Becoming a Physical Therapist:
The Complete Guide

Becoming a Physical Therapist: The Complete Guide

Frank Gregory

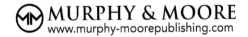

MURPHY & MOORE
www.murphy-moorepublishing.com

Becoming a Physical Therapist: The Complete Guide
Frank Gregory
ISBN: 978-1-63987-809-3 (Hardback)

Ⓜ MURPHY & MOORE

Murphy & Moore Publishing
1 Rockefeller Plaza,
New York City,
NY 10020, USA

Cataloging-in-Publication Data

Becoming a physical therapist : the complete guide / Frank Gregory.
    p. cm.
Includes bibliographical references and index.
ISBN 978-1-63987-809-3
1. Physical therapists--Vocational guidance. 2. Physical therapy--Vocational guidance. I. Gregory, Frank.
RM705 .B43 2023
615.82--dc23

Table of Contents

VI   Contents

Permissions

Index

Preface

Physical therapy is a healthcare profession concerned with the application of manual therapy, biomechanics or kinesiology, exercise therapy, electrotherapy, etc. to treat impairments and promote mobility and function. The purpose of physical therapy is to enhance a patient's quality of life through the effective diagnosis, prognosis, intervention and education of patients. Some specialization areas of physical therapy are cardiovascular and pulmonary physiotherapy, geriatric, integumentary, orthopedic and neurological physical therapy, among others. The outcomes of physical therapy typically include the management of pain, ability to perform activities of daily living, management of depression, etc. This book is a compilation of topics that discuss the most vital concepts in the field of physical therapy. Different approaches, evaluations and methodologies have been included in this book. It aims to serve as a resource guide for students and experts alike.

To facilitate a deeper understanding of the contents of this book a short introduction of every chapter is written below:

Chapter 1- Physical therapy, also called physiotherapy, is a health care profession, which uses kinesiology or biomechanics, exercise therapy, manual therapy and electrotherapy for the management of physical impairments and promotion of mobility and function of the body. It is aimed at improving the quality of life for a patient. This is an introductory chapter, which discusses about the various roles and responsibilities of a physical therapist and the ways to start a career in physical therapy.

Chapter 2- Physical therapy is a vast field and physical therapists may specialize in one or more areas. Some commonly recognized physical therapy specializations include geriatric physical therapy, orthopedic physical therapy, pediatric physical therapy, etc. This chapter explores the diverse areas of physical therapy and provides a step-by-step guide to begin careers in these domains.

Chapter 3- Physical therapy services can be provided as primary care treatment along with other medical services. This chapter has been carefully written to provide an easy understanding of the varied physical therapy treatments for the management of muscular dystrophy, arthritis, osteoporosis and for recovery from surgery, stroke, sports injuries, back pain, etc.

Chapter 4- Massage is the manual manipulation of the body using fingers, hands, knees, elbows, feet or any device. It is done for the treatment of stress or pain and for general health and well-being. The topics elaborated in this chapter will help in gaining a better perspective about the significant aspects of physical therapy and the ways to start a massage therapy business and become a massage therapist. It also explores the techniques of delivering effective hot stone massage, full body massage, leg massage, etc.

Finally, I would like to thank the entire team involved in the inception of this book for their valuable time and contribution. This book would not have been possible without their efforts. I would also like to thank my friends and family for their constant support.

Frank Gregory

CHAPTER 1

Physical Therapist: Career Prospects

Physical therapy, also called physiotherapy, is a health care profession, which uses kinesiology or biomechanics, exercise therapy, manual therapy and electrotherapy for the management of physical impairments and promotion of mobility and function of the body. It is aimed at improving the quality of life for a patient. This is an introductory chapter, which discusses about the various roles and responsibilities of a physical therapist and the ways to start a career in physical therapy.

Physical Therapy

Physical therapy (PT) is care that aims to ease pain and help you function, move, and live better. You may need it to:

- Relieve pain
- Improve movement or ability
- Prevent or recover from a sports injury
- Prevent disability or surgery
- Rehab after a stroke, accident, injury, or surgery
- Work on balance to prevent a slip or fall
- Manage a chronic illness like diabetes, heart disease, or arthritis
- Recover after you give birth
- Control your bowels or bladder
- Adapt to an artificial limb
- Learn to use assistive devices like a walker or cane
- Get a splint or brace

Types

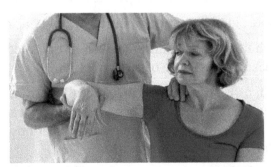

Physical therapy can help a patient regain movement or strength after an injury or illness.

As with any medical practice, a variety of therapies can be applied to treat a range of conditions.

Orthopedic physical therapy treats musculoskeletal injuries, involving the muscles, bones, ligaments, fascias, and tendons. It is suitable for medical conditions such as fractures, sprains, tendonitis, bursitis, chronic medical problems, and rehabilitation or recovery from orthopedic surgery. Patients may undergo treatment with joint mobilizations, manual therapy, strength training, mobility training, and other modalities.

Geriatric physical therapy can help older patients who develop conditions that affect their mobility and physical function, including arthritis, osteoporosis, Alzheimer's disease, hip and joint replacement, balance disorders, and incontinence. This type of intervention aims to restore mobility, reduce pain and increase physical fitness levels.

Neurological physical therapy can help people with neurological disorders and conditions such as Alzheimer's disease, brain injury, cerebral palsy, multiple sclerosis, Parkinson's disease, spinal cord injury, and stroke. Treatment may aim to increase limb responsiveness, treat paralysis, and reverse increase muscles strength by reducing muscle atrophy.

Cardiovascular and pulmonary rehabilitation can benefit people affected by some cardiopulmonary conditions and surgical procedures. Treatment can increase physical endurance and stamina.

Pediatric physical therapy aims to diagnose, treat, and manage conditions that affect infants, children, and adolescents, including developmental delays, cerebral palsy, spina bifida, torticollis and other conditions that impact the musculoskeletal system.

Wound care therapy can help to ensure that a healing wound is receiving adequate oxygen and blood by way of improved circulation. Physical therapy may include the use of manual therapies, electric stimulation, compression therapy and wound care.

Vestibular therapy aims to treat balance problems that can result from inner ear conditions. Vestibular physical therapy involves a number of exercises and manual techniques that can help patients regain their normal balance and coordination.

Decongestive therapy can help to drain accumulated fluid in patients with lymphedema and other conditions that involve fluid accumulation.

Pelvic floor rehabilitation can help treat urinary or fecal incontinence, urinary urgency and pelvic pain in men and women as a result of injuries or surgery, or because of certain conditions.

Apart from physical manipulation, physical therapy treatment may involve:
- Ultrasound, to promote blood flow and healing by heating the tendons, muscles, and tissues.
- Phonophoresis, which uses ultrasound to deliver certain medications such as topical steroids. This can decrease the presence of inflammation.
- Electrical stimulation, or E-stim, which uses topical electrodes on the skin to reduce pain and increase functional capabilities. One type of E-stim is transcutaneous electrical nerve stimulation (TENS). At times, anti-inflammatory medications are used with certain E-stim modalities and is referred to as iontophoresis.
- Heat, moist heat and cold therapy.

- Light therapy, in which special lights and lasers are used to treat certain medical conditions.

Physical Therapist

A physical therapist's main job is to help people who have been injured or who are disabled restore physical mobility and joint function through targeted exercise. Most therapists work one-on-one with patients, and typically design stretches and programs specific to the injuries or concerns at issue. They often work in conjunction with hospitals or nursing homes, and are usually considered to be members of the medical or healthcare profession.

Patients usually seek physical therapy for defined reasons. A person who has a broken arm may seek short-term therapy in order to re-teach muscles how to do things like hold a pencil or type on a keyboard, for instance — activities that months in a cast may have hindered. Someone who has had a brain tumor removed or a foot amputated may require longer-term therapy, often spanning several years, in order to learn techniques for coping and building muscular strength. People who have been born with disabilities or physical handicaps may spend most of their lives in physical therapy as well. The day-to-day work of a physical therapist will necessarily depend on the needs of the patient, but the framework is usually the same no matter what.

Developing a Program

One of the most important parts of the job revolves around treatment plans. Therapists will typically meet with patients at least once in an informal, information-only capacity in order to learn more about what needs to be accomplished. This meeting often involves diagnostic stretches and sometimes even a cursory exam so that the therapist can get a sense of exactly what is going on. Review of medical records, charts, and other files often happens at this stage.

Next, the therapist will create a treatment program that starts small but builds on itself over time. The program will typically incorporate different exercises designed to help improve such things as range of motion, endurance, or motor skills. Use of weights and special stretching equipment is common, and massage therapy, traction, and heat or water therapy may also be incorporated in some circumstances. The therapist's job is to choose the exercises that are best suited for the patient's condition, then adjust them as needed to meet the end goals.

Helping Execute Exercises

Most physical therapy sessions last for an hour or more. During this time, therapists work directly with patients, first demonstrating the target exercise then monitoring to be sure it is being replicated properly. The therapist may adjust the intensity as required. Most of the time, he or she will also assign "homework" to patients in the form of at-home exercises that will build out of what was learned in the session.

Accessibility

Most physical therapists keep regular office hours, and are not usually on call the way many other medical professionals are. Still, most will give out their phone numbers or other contact information to patients, and may take after-hours calls or arrange emergency sessions as needed — though much of this depends on the specific practitioner.

Work Settings

Generally speaking, a physical therapist works in a hospital, nursing home, or other facility where medical treatment is provided, and usually coordinates care with physicians, nurses, psychologists, and occupational therapists. Therapists who work in hospitals often only provide short-term or intermediate care. People who are just coming out of surgery or who have recently been diagnosed with degenerative conditions are often the mainstay of the patient base in these settings. In nursing homes, veteran's recovery centers, and rehabilitation clinics, the relationships usually last longer.

An experienced physical therapist may also choose to work independently, often in a private office or as a consultant. Success in this sort of setting usually requires an established patient base, else a means of securing steady referrals; at the same time, though, it often allows much greater flexibility.

Training Requirements

The sort of education and licensing a physical therapist must receive varies by jurisdiction, though the burden is generally quite high. An undergraduate degree is almost universally required, and most places also mandate graduate work to at least the master's degree level. Graduates must typically pass a licensing or certification exam to begin seeing patients, which may or may not require a certain number of hours of fieldwork. Aspiring therapists often meet these burdens by completing internships or apprenticeships while in school.

How to Get Accepted into Physical Therapy Schools

Physical therapy (PT) is a demanding and competitive field. PT is the treatment of injury or pain through exercise or other corrective means. As part of the health profession, physical therapists must understand anatomy, biology, medical diagnosis, and physics, as well as the treatments for common ailments. These programs can be hard to get into, but there are some steps you can take to make you a perfect candidate to get accepted into PT schools.

Part 1. Getting Ready before you Apply

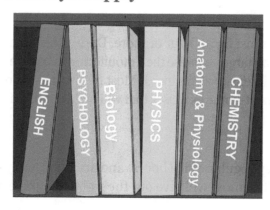

1. Take the right courses. If you know that you want to be in a health-related field like PT, you will have the opportunity to prove your interest and knowledge of the topics that are necessary for a PT degree. There are certain classes that are common requirement in your undergraduate career to make you the best candidate for a graduate program in PT. However, if you know the program you want to get into, make sure you check their specific requirements. Common courses include:

- Anatomy and physiology.
- All levels of biology.
- Chemistry.
- Physics.
- Psychology.
- English.

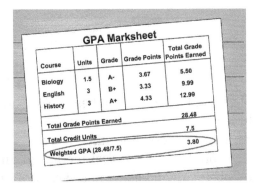

2. Maintain a high GPA. Since PT programs are so competitive, you need to make sure you look as good on paper as possible. Many or most PT schools use GPA as a highly weighed deciding factor for admission. The average GPA tends to be from 3.5 to 3.8.

- If you are having a hard time keeping your GPA up, think about tutoring, taking summer classes to devote more time to one class, or studying more. Since the programs are so competitive, your GPA needs to be as high as possible.

- Most PT programs have minimum GPA requirements, so check the program you are interested in to know what GPA to aspire to.

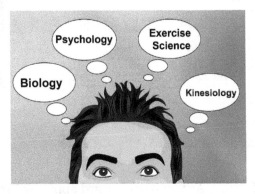

3. Worry less about your major. There is no specific major that PT schools look for when accepting

a student. However, since you are taking so many classes in the sciences, it is likely that a major that relates to science would make your degree easier on you. This way, you won't have to take too many classes outside the sciences to complete your major.

- There are some common majors, which include biology, psychology, exercise science, and kinesiology.

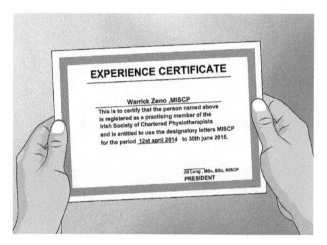

4. Get as much experience as possible. PT school is not easy. You should also be prepared to work hard in mentally and physically demanding classes. They are also highly competitive. Many schools choose only 30 students from over 200 to 600 applicants. You need to find ways to gain experience and work hard in order to be accepted into a physical therapy graduate program. Programs are typically looking for around 100 observational hours in a variety of settings.

- Find ways to get either volunteer or paid experience with a licensed physical therapist. Look into surrounding hospitals, physical therapy clinics, nursing homes, or other health-care establishments to find somewhere to get observational experience.

- These experiences are often required for program. Make sure your hours are verified by the licensed therapist you observe.

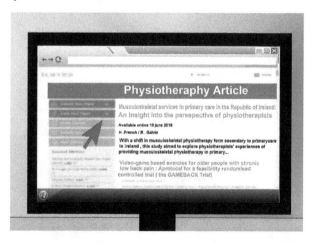

5. Keep up to date in the profession. As you work toward applying for PT school, you need to keep up to date in what is going on in the profession. Read current journals about the new practices that

are happening in the field. Learn about the specialties that the field offers so you know the options for your future and what you might want to specialize in.

- Figure out what about the field makes you want to pursue it. This will help you later when you are asked that kind of question in an admissions interview.

Part 2. Applying to a Program

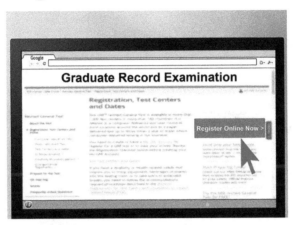

1. Take the Graduate Record Examination (GRE). When you are getting ready for applications, which is typically during your last year of your undergraduate degree, you need to take the GRE. The necessary score needed for your program will vary depending on the school that you apply to, but the scores range from 130-170 for Verbal and Quantitative Reasoning and 0 to 6 for Analytical Writing. You can arrange to take the GRE through your school or go to the Education Testing Service's website to find local testing centers.

- If you don't make the score that you need the first time around, there are preparatory classes you can take or books that you can get to help you increase your scores. There are also free test prep questions on the Educational Testing Service's website.

- Even if you haven't picked a school yet, you need to go ahead and take the GRE as soon as possible. The earlier you take it, the more time you have to retake it if you need higher scores.

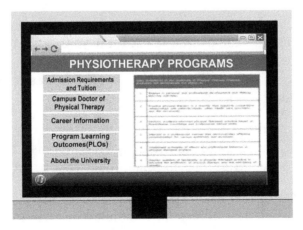

2. Find the right program for you. Before you apply, you need to make sure you have the right

program. When looking for the right school for you, look at the location of the school, the requirements for their PT program, the cost of the program, and any funding available. You also need to make sure that the program you are looking at is accredited in whatever country the school is in.

- Being accredited means that the country where the school is located recognizes it as a legitimate school that had the qualifications to provide you with the skills and coursework necessary for your degree.

- If you end up getting a degree at a school with no accreditation, your degree may be worthless.

- Each physical therapy school is slightly different. All schools will list their application requirements online or in their brochures. You may want to choose a school that aligns with your experience and qualifications.

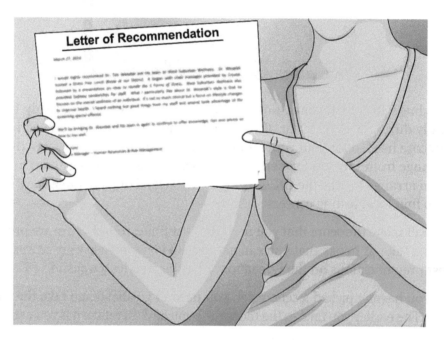

3. Ask for letters of recommendation. Almost all graduate programs require letters of recommendation from professors and professionals who can attest to your skills and merits as an individual, a student, and a future physical therapist. Try to make a great impression on the therapists you work with and the professors that you study under. Then, you can ask them for letters of recommendation that will be filled with praise for you.

- Typically, you will need at least three references when you apply to a physical therapy school. One of your references should be a physical therapist. You may be able to use the same references for all of the schools to which you choose to apply.

- Make sure whomever you ask knows you well enough to write you a great letter. You don't want to have mediocre letters of recommendation. You want to stand out against the rest of the thousands of students who apply to PT school each year.

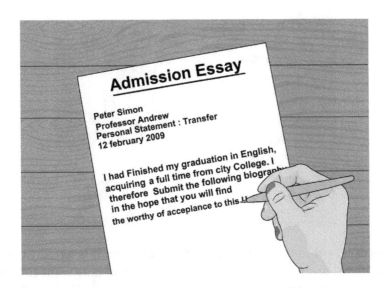

4. Write a great admission essay. Most applications will ask for an admissions essay. In your essay, you want to convince the admission board what makes you the best candidate for their school. Talk about your experiences in the field, the coursework that you completed to prepare you for an advanced degree, and how hard you will work in the program. Also express why you want to be a physical therapist, what the profession means to you, and what your future goals are.

- Essays can set you apart from other applicants who may have taken similar courses, have similar GPAs, and similar experience to you. The essay can make you more approachable and attractive to the admissions board.

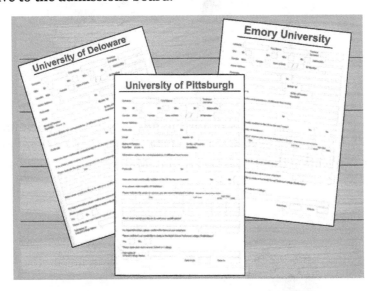

5. Apply to more than one school. Although each school most likely requires an application fee, you will increase your chances of getting into a school if you apply to three to five schools. If you get into more than one, you can choose which school you like best.

- Be meticulous in the application process. Avoid typos and ask your friends to proof your work. You may also ask for pointers from any physical therapists that you have worked for. Provide all the paperwork needed as requested, or your application may be overlooked.

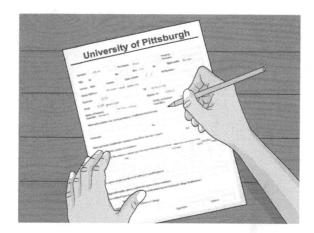

6. Keep trying. If you don't get in on your first try, don't give up. It is a really competitive field, and most programs turn away hundreds of students every year. You may want to broaden your base of schools that you apply to each year, in order to help your chances of being admitted.

- It may take a few tries to get in to the program you want, but don't lose hope.

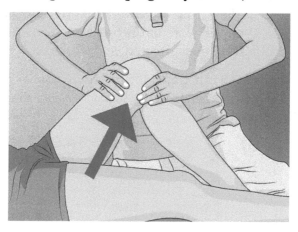

7. Get additional experience. While you wait for the next round of applications to come around, get more experience with licensed physical therapists to ensure that you have more experience and can add more to your application the next time around. Make sure you have varied settings such as rehab, outpatient, hospital and home health.

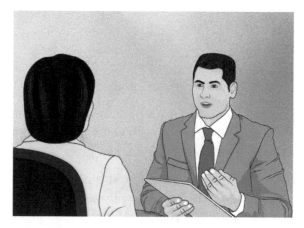

8. Practice your interviewing skills. Even if you do not get invited to interview for the school(s) you applied to, it is a good idea to practice mock interviews with seasoned interviewers. Preferably do this with a practicing P.T. that helps with the interviews, or the faculty that performs interviews. Their feedback will be invaluable. There are books on Amazon and Nook that delve further into the intricacies needed to make you a successful applicant.

How to Become a Physical Therapist

Physical therapists are medical professionals who specialize in helping patients both recover from and manage immobilities that result from injuries, illnesses, or surgeries. Physical therapy can be a very rewarding career, as it involves improving the overall quality of life for patients, as well as an average pay of $76,000 a year in the U.S.The demand for physical therapists is expected to increase by 39% from 2010 to 2020, making it one of the 30 fastest-growing careers in the United States. If you want to follow this rewarding career path, just follow these steps.

Method 1. Obtaining Licensure

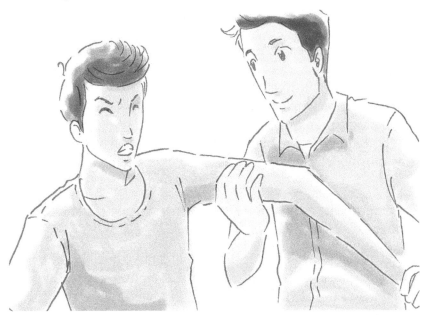

1. Make sure you have what it takes to be a physical therapist. Before you go into the educational program that is required for you to be a physical therapist, you should have a clear sense of what this career entails. If you want to obtain licensure and enjoy a career as a physical therapist, you should be prepared to do the following tasks:

- Diagnose your patients' dysfunctional movements by watching them move around and listening to their complaints and concerns.

- Devise an individualized plan for each patient, understanding the patients' goals.

- Use hands-on therapy, stretches, and exercises to help ease the pain of your patients and improve their mobility.

- Evaluate the progress of your patients and modify their treatment plans as needed.

- Tell your patients and their families about what they should expect as they recover from their injuries.

- Provide emotional support to your patients as you help them deal with their injuries.

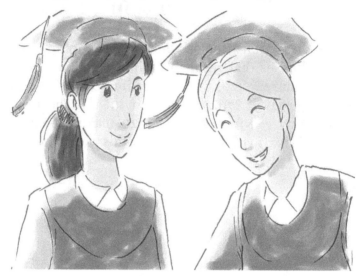

2. Get a bachelor's degree from a four-year university with a focus in science-based courses. While you don't necessarily have to obtain a BS (Bachelor of Science), the post-graduate program you apply to may have prerequisites in biology, chemistry, anatomy, or physiology. If you are currently an undergraduate and plan on becoming a physical therapist, talk to a counselor at your school to determine which courses you should be taking and whether you have chosen the right major.

- Common undergraduate majors for physical therapists include biology, psychology, and exercise science.

- You don't *have* to major in a science-based field, but you will have to take several courses that meet the prerequisite standards of your chosen post-graduate program. This means that you could major in Art History, Spanish, or another unrelated field, while taking the required courses to become a physical therapist.

- The average GPA for students accepted to physical therapy programs in 2011-2012 was 3.52, so be prepared to study rigorously during your time as an undergraduate.

- If you'd like to be a physical therapists' assistant, then you can earn an associates degree instead.

- There are a few physical therapy programs that allow students to enter directly after they graduate from high school. If you're interested in one of these freshman entry programs, you should look into them while you're still in high school.

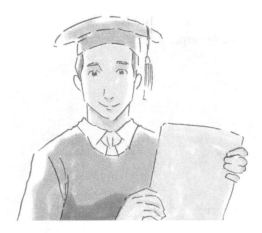

3. Obtain a post-graduate professional degree. Some post-graduate physical therapy programs offer a Doctor of Physical Therapy (DPT) degree, while others offer a Master of Physical Therapy (MPT) degree, though the DPT is far more common. Doctoral programs typically last for 3 years, while Master's programs last 2-3 years. The coursework covered includes anatomy, physiology, biomechanics, and neuroscience. Check out this link to find PT programs in your area.

- The program you choose may also involve completing a clinical rotation, during which you will gain hands-on experience working in the field.

- You may need to complete the Graduate Record Examination (GRE) to be accepted to the institute of your choice.

- The application process for post-graduate programs in physical therapy is competitive. To help your chances of acceptance, you should gain experience as a volunteer or a worker in a physical-therapy setting.

- You will need to provide 1-4 letters of reference when you apply to physical therapy programs, so make sure to build meaningful connections with your teachers and mentors before you apply.

- Make sure you choose the right PT program. Compare the programs based on their locations, areas of specialty, licensure passing rate, and financial aid packages.

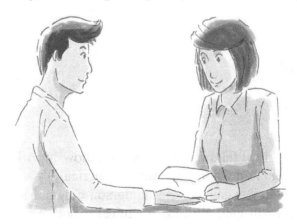

4. Obtain a license to practice physical therapy. Specific license requirements vary between states,

but most states require that prospective candidates pass the National Physical Therapy Examination (NPTE). Determine your state's requirements for physical therapy licenses.

Method 2. Succeeding in Your Career

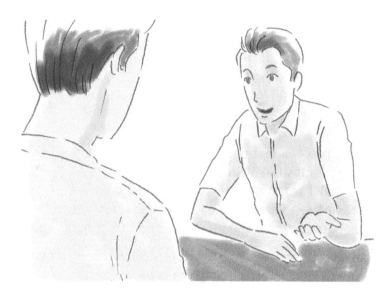

1. Consider applying to a clinical residency program. After you graduate from your program, you may consider applying to a residency program to gain additional training and as well as experience in specialized area of care. This will help improve your job prospects as well as give you more advancement in your field.

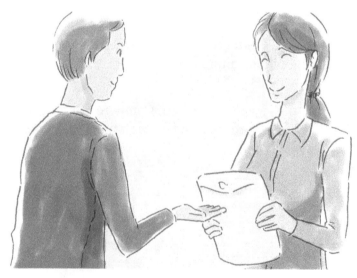

2. Consider applying for a clinical fellowship. A clinical fellowship will allow you to further your education in a specialized field and will offer a focused curriculum with advanced clinical and didactic instruction that can help you gain a better understanding of a subspecialty area of practice. You will have a mentor and will gain additional clinical experience and will work with enough patients to build your skills.

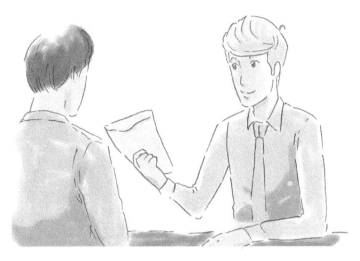

3. Find a job as a physical therapist. There are a variety of potential job settings for a physical therapist, including hospitals, clinics, outpatient facilities, homes, schools, and fitness centers. Check your local job listings to find availabilities in your area. Send your resume, cover letter, and whatever other information that your potential employer requests.

- Though not required, you will benefit from completing an internship or job working as a physical therapist's assistant (PAT) prior to becoming a physical therapist yourself. While working in this position, you will perform physical therapy on patients under the supervision of a certified professional.

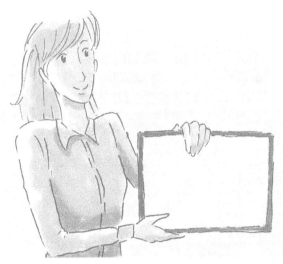

4. Get a board certification in a clinical specialty after you gain some work experience. Getting a board certification in a clinical specialty can help you gain expertise in a chosen field and will make you a more desirable job candidate and physical therapist. There are a variety of certifications that you can get, and you are not limited to choosing just one. Though physical therapists aren't required to get a board certification in a clinical specialty, this is a useful way to improve your education and skill set. Here are some common physical therapy certifications that may appeal to you:

- Cardiovascular and pulmonary therapy

- Clinical electrophysiology

- Geriatrics

- Neurology

- Orthopedics

- Pediatrics

- Sports

- Women's health

Method 3. Having the Qualities of a Physical Therapist

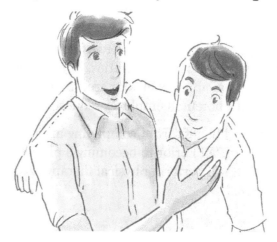

1. Be compassionate. It is important that physical therapists be warm, friendly individuals with strong communication skills, as the job requires constantly dealing with sick or injured patients. As a physical therapist, you will work with many people who suffer emotionally as well as physically because of their pain, and you will need to have a lot of empathy to help them heal and understand their injuries.

- It is important to also be patient, as many patients do not see immediate results and may require years of therapy.

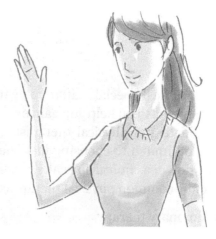

2. Have dexterity. Since physical therapy requires working with your hands, it is important to have strong manual dexterity. Physical therapists should also have strong enough arms to apply resistance to patients' limbs and help lift them up if necessary. You will need to be comfortable using your hands to help your patients do physical exercises as well as giving them manual therapy.

- Manual dexterity can be improved by activities like writing, sewing, knitting, and using a stress ball to strengthen hand muscles.

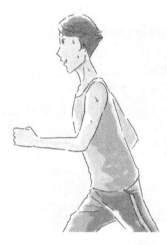

3. Be prepared to spend most of your time on your feet. Most physical therapists spent much of their time on their feet, not sitting in a chair. As a physical therapist, you'll need to move around to work with your patients and help them complete a variety of exercises. Therefore, you shouldn't be the type of person who sits down every chance he gets and should actually enjoy physical activity.

- You should also be physically fit not only to be able to work with your patients more easily, but also to inspire confidence in your patients. Your patients will want to work with someone who cares about his own physical fitness, too.

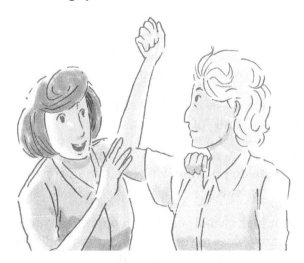

4. Have strong people skills. You should not only know how to be compassionate toward your patients, but you should be "a people person," and should be comfortable interacting with your

patients, making them laugh, and keeping up a good rapport as you work together. You should also be able to speak openly to your patients about their treatment programs and listen to their concerns about the therapy.

How to Get a Doctorate in Physical Therapy

If you want to become a practicing physical therapist in the United States, you will need to obtain a doctor of physical therapy (DPT) degree. Earning this degree involves completing three years of coursework beyond a bachelor's degree and meeting the chosen university's requirement for hands-on practice with patients. The earlier you begin preparing for this program, the easier it will be to get in.

Part 1. Fulfilling the Prerequisite Requirements

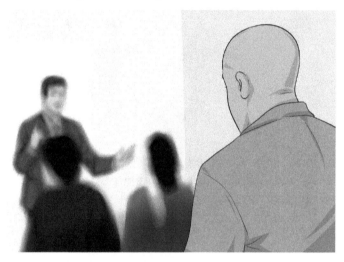

1. Start focusing your studies in high school. If you are still a high school student, you can start working right now to improve your chances of being accepted into a DPT program in a few years. Choosing classes that relate to your future career and getting the best grades possible is an excellent way to start.

- Take as many science classes as you can in high school, especially AP classes. The more fundamental knowledge you have, the better prepared you will be for college-level classes.

- Don't neglect your other classes in favor of science classes. It's important to be well-rounded and have good grades in all your courses.

- A high GPA and good SAT or ACT scores will improve your chances of being accepted into an excellent undergraduate program, which will in turn prepare you for the graduate program that you want to pursue.

- You can also use your high school years as an opportunity to shadow professional physical therapists. Reach out to offices in your area and try to find a therapist who would be willing to let you observe their daily routine. This will give you a good idea of what it is really like to be a physical therapist.

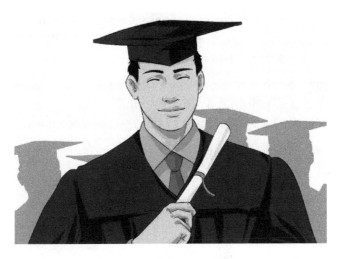

2. Complete a bachelor's degree program. In order to be accepted into a doctoral program in physical therapy, you will first need to complete an undergraduate degree. All doctoral programs have different prerequisite requirements, so it's a good idea to review the requirements at several schools before choosing your undergraduate major. In general, you will be required to take undergraduate courses in science fields such as biology, chemistry, anatomy, and physiology.

- Especially relevant majors include biology, kinesiology, and exercise science, although you may have other options as well, depending on what programs are offered at your undergraduate school and what graduate school you hope to attend.

- If you are still in high school and you are certain that you want to pursue a doctorate degree in physical therapy, you may want to look into applying to a guaranteed admission program. These programs admit students as college freshmen for a six-year program that encompasses an undergraduate degree and a doctorate degree without the need to apply separately for the doctoral program.

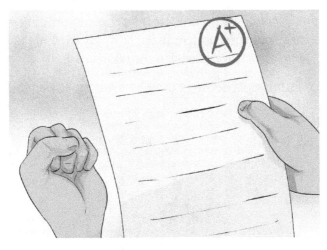

3. Work hard for good grades. Most reputable DPT programs are highly competitive, and undergraduate GPAs are heavily weighed by graduate program admissions officers, so it is extremely important to keep your grades as high as possible. Stay focused on your goals throughout your undergraduate years and maintain the highest GPA possible.

- If you are struggling with your undergraduate classes, get help as soon as possible. Talk to your professors about what you can do to improve your grades or find out if there are peer tutoring services available at your university.

- Avoid overloading yourself with classes as an undergraduate if it causes your grades to slip. For example, if you can maintain a 3.6 GPA while taking 15 credits, but only a 3.2 while taking 18 credits, it may be wise to stick to the 15-credit course load.

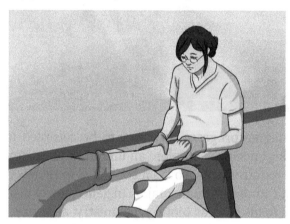

4. Gain experience in the field. Having some kind of experience in the physical therapy field or a closely related field can greatly improve your chances of being admitted to a doctoral program. You can gain experience by getting a part-time job, completing an internship program, or even volunteering.

- Many programs will require that you complete observation hours before a DPT program. If this is required for the program that you will be applying for, make the most of this experience! Try to form a good relationship with the physical therapists you shadow, as you will probably need them to write recommendation letters for you.

- In addition to helping you get into a doctoral program, gaining experience at the undergraduate level will also help you confirm that you enjoy working in the field, and it also may help you choose a specialty that you wish to pursue.

- Having experience in multiple settings may be even more beneficial, so seek out as many relevant opportunities as possible.

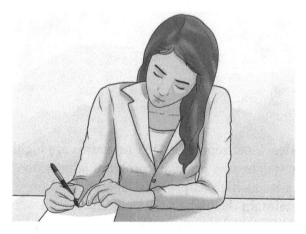

5. Take the Graduate Record Examination. The Graduate Record Examination (GRE) is a test that is required for admission to most graduate programs, including DPT programs. Scores are valid for five years, so you can take it any time during your undergraduate studies. Be sure to prepare for this test and do as well as you can, as GRE scores are heavily weighed by admissions officers.

- The GRE is a standardized test that consists of three sections: verbal reasoning, quantitative reasoning, and analytical writing.

- Check online to find out what GRE scores you will need to be accepted into various DPT programs. Many schools post this information on their websites. If they don't post a minimum required score, they may post the average score of accepted applicants.

- You can retake the GRE if your score is not as high as you hoped it would be. The earlier you take the exam, the more chances you will have to retake it before you have to submit your applications to DPT programs.

- When you take the GRE, you can select to have your scores automatically sent to the schools that you plan on applying to. If you don't do this before you take the test, you will need to contact the company that administers the exam to have your scores sent to each school.

Part 2. Applying to a Doctorate Program

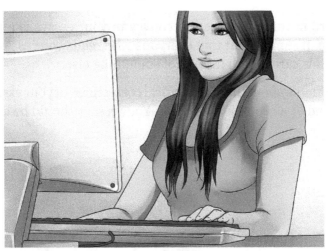

1. Decide which schools you will apply to. In general, it's a good idea to apply to several different DPT programs, as admissions are typically very competitive. Before applying, take a look at the admissions requirements online. If you are unsure if you will be accepted into the programs that you are most interested in, consider applying to several "safe" schools with less stringent admissions requirements as well.

- When looking at schools, it is extremely important to ensure that they are accredited by the Commission on Accreditation in Physical Therapy Education (CAPTE). In order to sit for the exam that is required to obtain a license to practice physical therapy, you will need to graduate from an accredited program.

- Some factors to consider when selecting the right school for you are graduation and employment rates, location, cost, and program size.

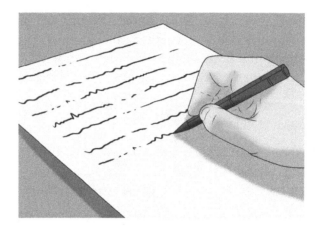

2. Write your admissions essays. Most applications will require that you write at least one essay. Even if writing is not your strong point, be sure to take your time and write quality essays. Always read the requirements carefully to make sure that you answer all aspects of the question that is being asked and adhere to the required word count.

- If you are asked to write essays on different topics for different schools, make sure your essay really fits the topic. Don't just tweak an essay that you used for another application if it doesn't fit!

- The most important thing you need to convey in your essays is a passion for the field of physical therapy. It's important that everyone who reads your essays understand why you want to pursue this career path instead of something else.

- If you have any doubts about the grammatical correctness of your essays, have them checked by a trusted friend or a professional editor. Your essays should be as polished as possible!

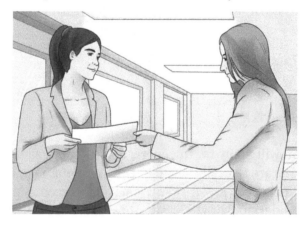

3. Obtain letters of recommendation. Letters of recommendation are also a very important component of your application. Each program will have specific requirements for letters of recommendation, but they should generally come from college professors and/or professionals in the physical therapy field.

- Ask professors who can speak to your ability to excel in a science-heavy curriculum and hands-on work with patients. The better the professors know you, the better their recommendation letters will be, so take some time to forge relationships with some of your professors.

- You may also need to obtain at least one letter of recommendation from a licensed physical therapist. This can be an individual that you shadowed during your observation hours, or an individual who you worked for in another capacity. These letters should highlight your aptitude for the field of physical therapy.

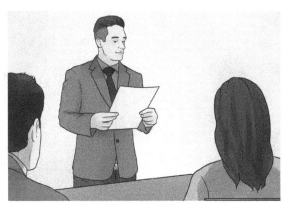

4. Complete the applications. Once you have gathered all of the required materials, complete the application for each DPT program that you wish to apply for. Most programs now use The Physical Therapy Centralized Application Service's online application, which makes it easy to apply to multiple programs.

- Be sure to submit all required documents before the application deadline. This includes transcripts, letters of recommendation, GRE scores, and any other documentation requested by the program.

- If there are multiple application deadlines, try to submit your application before the first deadline, as this may increase your chances of being accepted.

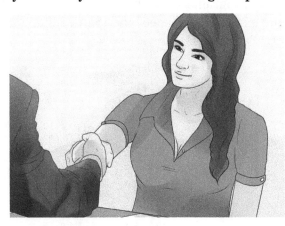

5. Attend in-person interviews. Some programs interview you in person to gauge your capacity for grasping the curriculum and working with people in a healthcare setting. If you are asked to attend an interview, use this as another opportunity to convey your passion for the field of physical therapy to the admissions committee.

- Even if you don't have an interview, it's a good idea to visit each school that you are interested in and talk with the faculty. This will give you a much better idea of which school is the best fit for you.

Part 3. Completing a Doctorate Program

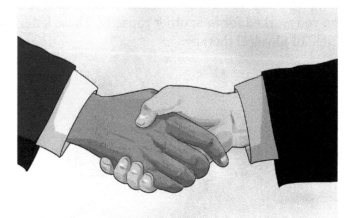

1. Accept an offer. Once you've applied to DPT programs, you will need to wait for your decision letters before making any further plans. If you are only accepted into one program, you will have an easy decision, but if you are accepted into multiple programs, you will need to carefully consider which is the best fit for you.

- There are three possible outcomes of an application to a DPT program: you may be accepted outright, you may be rejected outright, or you may be wait-listed. If you are wait-listed, this means that you will be given a spot in the program only if enough of the accepted candidates decline their offers. You may have to wait some time to find out if you are accepted into these programs.

- If you didn't get into any programs, don't give up! You may want to consider spending the next year gaining more clinical experience, and then applying to different programs.

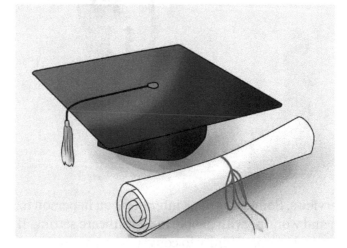

2. Complete the coursework. Most DPT programs take three years to complete. As a doctoral student, you can expect to spend about 80% of your time in the classroom and laboratory studying topics such as biology, physiology, behavioral sciences, finance, ethics, and sociology, and various evidence-based practices.

- It's a good idea to work closely with your academic adviser to plan out your coursework.

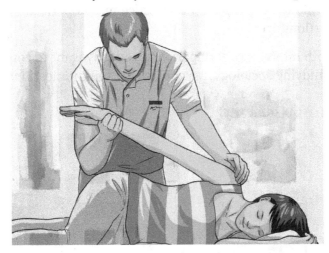

3. Fulfill the clinical fieldwork requirements. In addition to classroom work, you will be required to complete clinical fieldwork, which will constitute approximately 20% of your study time. This fieldwork will give you the opportunity to work with patients in a clinical setting under the supervision of licensed physical therapists. Each program has its own set of requirements.

- During your fieldwork, you will essentially be an intern, working in a clinical setting such as a hospital or private office under the supervision of a licensed physical therapist. You will both observe your mentor and be observed as you interact with and treat patients.

- You may be required to present a case study report based on a specific case that you encountered during your fieldwork.

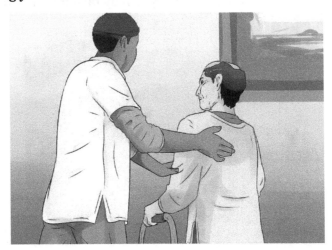

4. Hone your personal skills. In addition to learning about the science behind physical therapy, you will need to learn how to interact with patients in order to be a successful physical therapist. Use your field work during graduate school as an opportunity to improve your communication skills.

- You will need to be especially careful about explaining things to your patients in ways that they can understand. Using too much industry jargon will only confuse them.

- Consider asking your fellow students or supervisors for feedback on how you can improve the way that you interact with patients. Practice makes perfect, so do your best to implement their suggestions every day.

- If you struggle with interacting with patients, you may want to consider taking some additional courses. Studying sociology, psychology, or communications may help.

Part 4. Advancing your Career

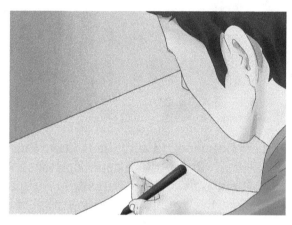

1. Take the National Physical Therapy Examination (NPTE). After you complete your doctoral program, the first step towards obtaining a license to practice physical therapy is to pass the NPTE. This is a computer-based multiple-choice exam that will test you on your knowledge of the practice of physical therapy.

- If you do not pass the NPTE the first time, you may take it up to three times per year until you pass.

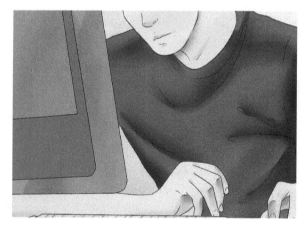

2. Fulfill the other requirements for licensure in your state. Each state in the United States sets its own requirements for obtaining a license to practice physical therapy. After you pass the NPTE, you may need to take some additional steps in order to obtain the license. Check with your state for more details.

- You may have to take additional exams beyond the• NPTE. These exams may include questions about the laws that are specific to the practice of physical therapy in your state.

- You may also have to pass a criminal background check in order to be granted a license.

- Many states also require that physical therapists complete continuing education requirements in order to renew their licenses.

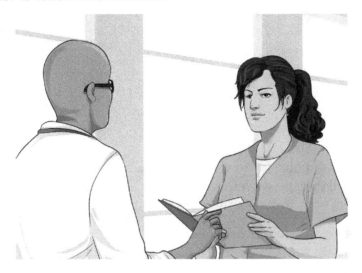

3. Complete a clinical residency or fellowship program. If you want to gain even more knowledge and skills beyond what you acquired during your DPT program, you may choose to pursue a clinical residency or fellowship program. These programs are designed for licensed physical therapists who wish to develop their knowledge in a specific area of clinical practice.

- Residency programs allow physical therapists to continue practicing under the guidance and mentorship of more experienced physical therapists. Fellowship programs include classroom instruction in addition to clinical work.

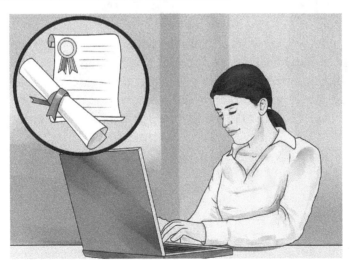

4. Pursue a specialty certification. Once you are licensed, you will also have the option to pursue board certification in a sub-specialty of physical therapy. This is not a requirement to be a licensed physical therapist, but it can help you earn respect in your field and gain more specific knowledge.

- Specialty areas include geriatrics, pediatrics, orthopedics, pulmonary and cardiovascular, women's health, neurology, clinical electrophysiology, and sports physical therapy.

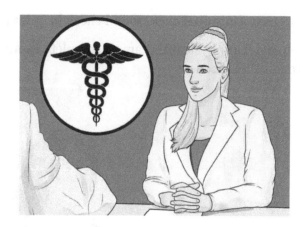

5. Make professional connections. If you want to continue growing your career and learning more about the field of physical therapy, it's important to stay connected to other industry professionals. There are many different ways to stay in the know, so take advantage of them.

- You can join professional organizations, such as the American Physical Therapy Association, which will help you stay up-to-date on the latest industry trends.

- You can subscribe to industry publications to stay informed. These may focus on a specific specialty of physical therapy or be more general, and many are available online for easy access.

- You may also wish to attend periodic conferences for physical therapists. This will give you the opportunity to learn about what other professionals in the field are doing and to network.

How to Become a Physical Therapist Assistant

Physical therapist assistants (PTAs) work as part of a dynamic healthcare team. Assistants help physical therapists maintain therapy facilities and monitor patient progress, while also helping patients by assisting them on difficult movements and instructing them on how to use walking aids. The PTA field is one of the fastest growing careers in health care, with even more jobs projected to open up over the next few years. Learn how to take the first steps toward this rewarding and challenging field.

Part 1. Getting an Education

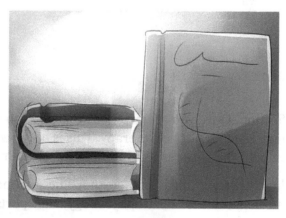

1. Take relevant high school courses. If you're considering a career as a physical therapy assistant, it's never too early to start preparing yourself. Taking advanced classes in biology, chemistry, and algebra - and earning high grades - can help you get into a college program that specializes in physical therapy assistance. Some PTA programs require a minimum average in algebra, so studying hard early on can help you go far in this field.

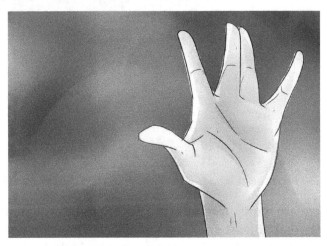

2. Consider volunteer work. Though it's not a requirement for getting into a PTA program, volunteering at a hospital or other health care facility will look great on a resume, and can help you decide if this career is right for you.

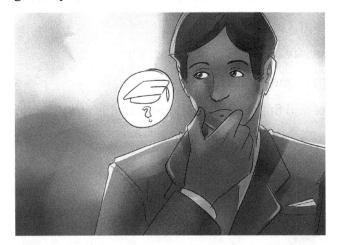

3. Find an accredited program. The minimum college educational requirement for PTAs is an associate's degree in physical therapist assistant education. It's important to ensure that the program you choose is accredited if you want to pursue a career as a PTA.

- In the United States, the only agency that grants accreditation status is the Commission on Accreditation in Physical Therapy Education (CAPTE). You can find a database of CAPTE-accredited programs on the American Physical Therapy Association's website.

- In Canada, accreditation is granted by the Physiotherapy Education Accreditation Canada (PEAC), and all physiotherapy programs across Canada are currently accredited by the PEAC.

- If you're unsure of the accrediting board in your place of residence, you can find out by searching online for the PTA accreditation board in your region.

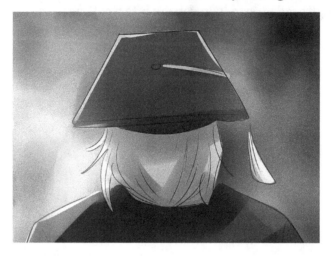

4. Get an education. There are many programs in PTA offered throughout the world. Accredited programs should mandate that at least 1/4 of a candidate's education be spent in a clinical environment. Other factors to consider while choosing a program include:

- The structure and curriculum of a program

- The types of clinical education and training opportunities offered through a program

- Available facilities at a program

- The licensure pass rate of students in a program

- Post-graduate employment statistics

- Cost of attendance and financial aid options available at a program

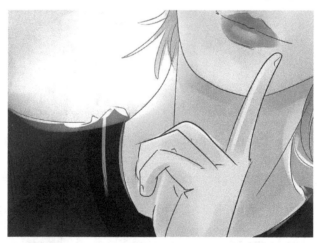

5. Consider an internship. Undertaking an internship while you're studying to become a PTA can drastically improve a candidate's chances of gaining employment after graduation. That's because internships provide interns with hands-on training and experience, and allows the intern to make valuable connections with experts in the field.

Part 2. Getting Licensed or Certified

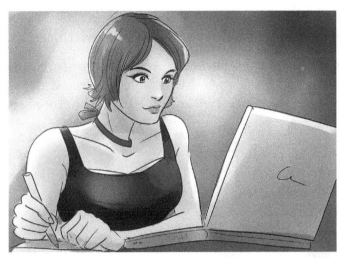

1. Study for the National Physical Therapy Exam. Candidates in the United States who have completed the educational requirements must pass the National Physical Therapy Exam, which is administered by Federation of State Boards of Physical Therapy (FSBPT). Candidates may not take the exam more than three times in a 12 month period, and may not take the exam more than six times overall.

- Study guides and practice exams can be found online on the FSBPT website.

- If you live outside the United States, you can learn about license/certification requirements in your country by searching online for your regional PT board.

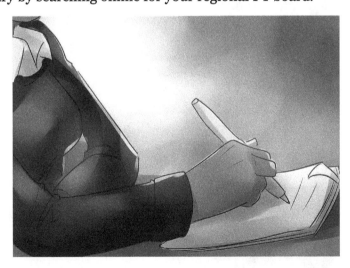

2. Take the National Physical Therapy Exam. The exam consists of 200 questions, broken up into four sections with 50 questions each. Candidates have four hours to complete the exam, and should arrive at least 30 minutes before the exam time.

- Exams are administered by Prometric at designated testing facilities on fixed dates throughout the year. Candidates can register for the exam and find testing locations and test dates on the FSBPT website, under "Registration Process".

- The exam for PTAs costs $70, payable to Prometric at the time candidates register for the exam.

- Bring two forms of ID, one of which must be a valid, government-issued photo ID.

- Each section of the exam contains both scored and un-scored (pretest) questions. Candidates have no way of knowing which questions are scored and which are un-scored, so candidates should treat each question as though it will be scored.

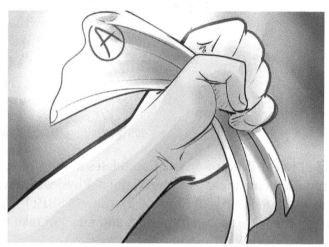

3. Pass the exam. Candidates will be issued a score on a scale between 200 and 800. In order to pass the exam, candidates must have earned a score of 600 or higher. Scores are reported to a candidate's jurisdiction roughly five business days after the exam, and scores will be made available for free to all candidates after 10 business days. Scores can be found and downloaded on the FSBPT website, under the "Status of My Request" tab.

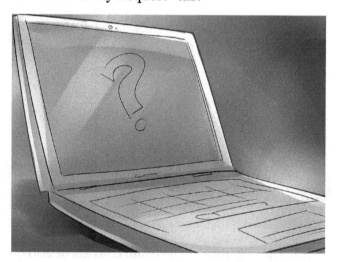

4. Learn your state's requirements. In addition to the National Physical Therapy Exam, some states also require candidates to complete and pass an additional state-wide exam and undergo a criminal background check. You can find your state's requirements by going to the Federation of State Boards of Physical Therapy website and clicking on "Licensing Authorities Contact Information".

Part 3. Knowing What's Expected of a PTA

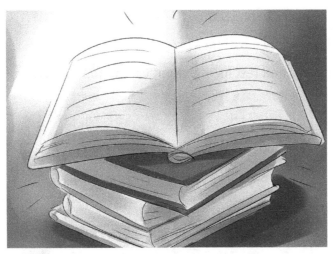

1. Learn about continuing education requirements. Some states require PTAs to take continuing education courses in order to maintain licensure. These requirements vary from state to state, and may not be required in jurisdictions outside the US. Contact your state/local board to learn about the licensing requirements in your region.

- PTAs can find a list of continuing education courses offered by the American Physical Therapy Association by visiting http://learningcenter.apta.org/Student/Catalogue/Catalogue. aspx.

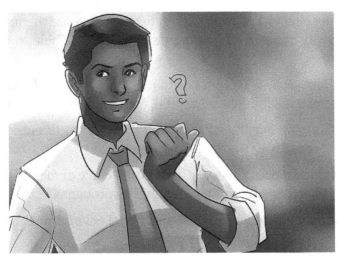

2. Know the duties of a PTA. PTAs work in a dynamic field, and the particulars of a PTAs work requirements will vary depending on the PTA's chosen work setting. Some common requirements of PTAs include:

- Working with physical therapists (PTs) and following a PT's orders
- Assisting patients with exercises and stretches
- Lifting or carrying patients as needed

- Massaging and bathing patients

- Applying heat/ice packs to patients

- Monitoring and recording a patient's progress

- Reporting all findings and results of patient care to the supervising physical therapist

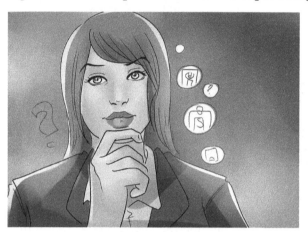

3. Choose a work setting. PTAs typically work in a clinical setting, but there are a number of work settings within hospitals, schools, and private PT offices.

- Acute Care - PTAs work with short-term patients in a hospital setting. PTAs only work with the patient until he or she is capable of being discharged from the hospital.

- Rehabilitation Hospital - PTAs work with patients for intense therapy lasting three or more hours each day with the goal of helping patients become able to administer self care at home.

- Sub-Acute Rehabilitation - PTAs work with patients at a special hospital facility with similar goals to those of a rehabilitation hospital, but with less-intense sessions.

- Extended Care/Nursing Facility - PTAs work primarily with elderly patients in a facility designed for long-term care.

- Outpatient/Private Practice Clinic - patients visit a clinic or facility to work with PTAs, primarily focusing on orthopedic and neuromuscular problems.

- School - PTAs work with students in an educational environment.

- Wellness/Prevention/Sports/Fitness - PTAs work with patients with an overall focus on physical wellbeing and injury prevention.

- Home Care - PTAs visit patients at the patient's home, residential facility, or even hospital room. Home care PTAs primarily work with patients who are senior citizens and/or patients who have significant disabilities.

- Hospice - PTAs work with patients who suffer from incurable ailments, with a focus on managing pain and increasing functional abilities for as long as possible.

- Occupational Environments - PTAs work to help improve safety and productivity in a work setting and help patients regain the strength to return to work.

- Government Settings - PTAs work with both civilians and military personnel at local, state, and federal agencies, including the Veteran's Health Administration and the Indian Health Service.

- Research Centers - PTAs may work with physical therapists and other medical professionals on research to increase knowledge of physical therapy and find ways to improve patient care outcomes in all settings.

Part 4. Finding a PTA Job

1. Build your resume. The most important things on a resume are your education, experience, and qualifications.

- List your education first, in reverse-chronological order, with your most recent degree at the top.

- Consider listing any relevant coursework that would qualify you for a position.

- List any relevant employment experience in reverse-chronological order.

- Summarize your background and experience (including any internships or volunteer work) under the "qualifications" heading.

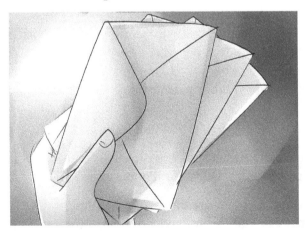

2. Apply to jobs. You can find open positions by searching relevant PTA job boards, or by looking at

the employment section on local hospitals' websites. Find PTA job boards in your area by searching online for physical therapy associations near you.

- You may also want to consider sending your resume and cover letter directly to a human resources representative at a facility you'd like to work at. Even if there are no openings at the time, they may keep you in mind for future openings.

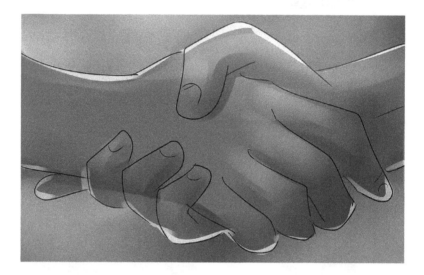

3. Make connections. Many PTAs get their first job by making connections during an internship. If you worked an internship or performed any volunteer work related to your field, contact the internship coordinator or a person of seniority at the facility where you worked and let them know that you're interested in working for them.

How to Start a Physical Therapy Business

Physical therapy practices are part of an ever-changing health sciences industry. Physical therapy has become one of the main ways that doctors help patients to overcome injury, regain mobility and learn proper body mechanics. After years of working as a physical therapist, you may decide you want to own your own practice. You should evaluate your motivation, financial health and competition to determine if you can feasibly start a successful physical therapy business. It is important to be slow and deliberate with your plans, because, like any small business, it will face many challenges on the road to profitability. Learn how to start a physical therapy business.

Steps

1. Research the market before deciding to start a physical therapy business. There is a lot of competition in physical therapy practices. Consider it a feasible idea if one of the following are true:

- You offer specialty services that are under represented in your town. This may include pediatric, geriatric, pool therapy, joint, sport or other physical therapy specializations. If you research your competition and find it is small or caters to a different niche market, then you will have an advantage.

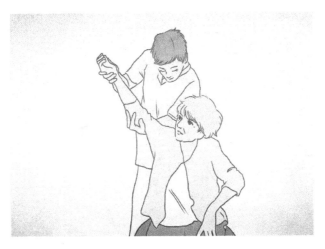

- You plan to hire other specialty physical therapists or provide other underrepresented services, such as pool therapy or massage.

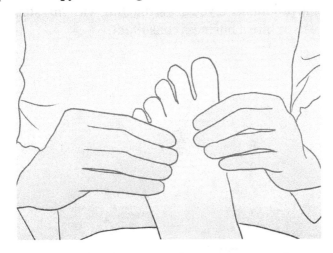

- You want to start a franchise of an established Physical Therapy clinic. If you currently work for a bustling physical therapy practice, or you know of 1 that is open to expansion, schedule a meeting to discuss starting a franchise in another location. You can use the reputation and network that is already created, while still running your own business.

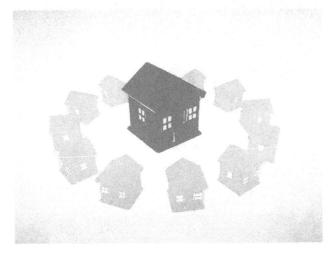

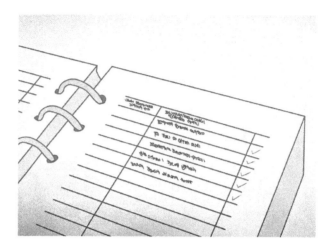

2. Create a business plan. Within the plan, you should explain the business objective, plans to raise financial support, competition, management, marketing, a calendar and the time period in which the business should become profitable. If you are struggling with this step, get help from a chapter of the small business bureau or hire a business consultant.

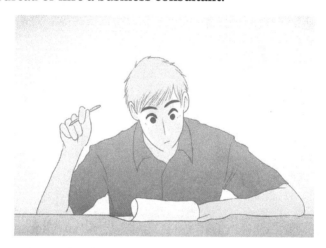

3. Leave your previous position on a positive note. Starting your own practice can be contentious because you are likely to be competition for your current employers. Explain the reasons you feel it is necessary to start your practice and your desire to remain on good terms.

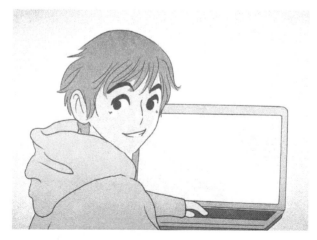

4. Create an account on the American Physical Therapy Association website. Visit their section on starting a practice at apta.org/PracticeOwnership. You can find excellent advice for choosing a structure, leasing space and more.

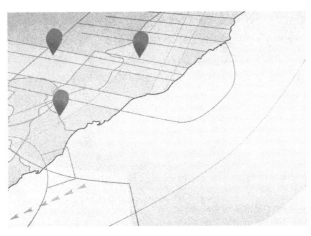

5. Choose a location for your physical therapy practice. As soon as you have secured funding, or while you are in the process, you should look for a location with the nearby demographic you often treat. Consider being away from your competition but close to a medical facility.

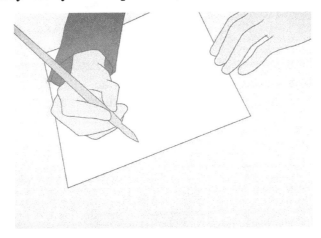

6. Begin filling out and filing all the necessary paperwork for your physical therapy practice. There are a number of things that are required by the state or country to ensure you are doing business within the legal framework. This includes topic of incorporation, partnerships and tax documents.

- Choose a name that is easy to remember. If you plan to have a solo practice, you may just want to use your full name. If you plan to hire more physical therapists, you may choose a general name that states the purpose of your clinic. Fill out and file a "Doing Business As" form with the county or state.

- Make sure your personal physical therapy license is up to date with the state. Then, apply for a business license in your county and state.

- File your incorporation documents with the state. Also, apply for an Employment Identification Number (EIN) with the Internal Revenue Service (IRS). This will allow you to hire employees and withhold income tax.

- Apply for insurance. This may include practice liability insurance, malpractice insurance, property insurance and health insurance for employees. You may hire a small business consultant to help research your options.

- Join physical therapy networks, such as PTPN, if you want to accept insurance. It is a good idea for many practices. You can receive insurance contracts through these networks. This usually means receiving a listing on their website and payment, in exchange for some substantial discounts when you receive payment from the insurance company.

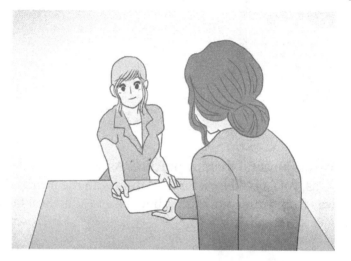

7. Hire competent and trustworthy staff for your business. After you secure a location and file paperwork, you will begin forming the structure of your office. Identify and fill the places according to the space, number of physical therapists you want, assistants and other staff.

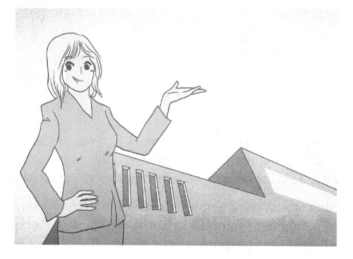

8. Begin marketing your business as soon as you are able to. As well as doing television, radio and print advertising, you should begin marketing your specialty services to local doctors, clinics and hospitals. Referrals from friends, family and medical practices are likely to provide the majority of your patients.

- Set your rates according to their going rate in your state. You may decide to give discounts for new clients in the first 6 months, to help your practice get started.

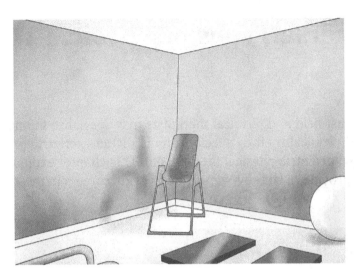

9. Buy equipment and set up your office. As identified by your business plan, starting a physical therapy practice requires good start up capital because you need a location and a good amount of equipment. Make investments in durable, essential workout, massage and other equipment.

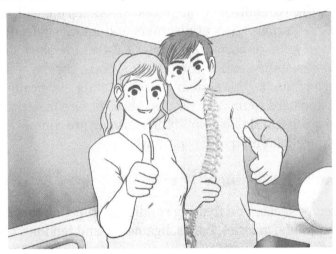

10. Be persistent. It will take a few years of networking, marketing, overtime and strong management to make a new physical therapy business a success. If you are determined to see the business to a successful stage, then you are more likely to be able to handle the obstacles that you face.

CHAPTER 2

Diverse Types of Physical Therapists

Physical therapy is a vast field and physical therapists may specialize in one or more areas. Some commonly recognized physical therapy specializations include geriatric physical therapy, orthopedic physical therapy, pediatric physical therapy, etc. This chapter explores the diverse areas of physical therapy and provides a step-by-step guide to begin careers in these domains.

Orthopedic Physical Therapy

Orthopedic physical therapy includes treatment of the musculoskeletal system (which is made up of the muscles and bones of the body) that has been subject to injury or trauma. This includes sprains, strains, post fracture, post surgery and repetitive injuries. The areas of the body include the neck and back as well the extremities. Orthopedics is a branch of medicine focused on the muscular and skeletal systems. Various types of disorders and injuries affecting our muscles, bones, and joints while discovering the important role physical therapy plays in managing orthopedic conditions. The musculoskeletal system is composed of bone, cartilage, ligaments, muscle, tendons, synovium, bursae and fascia. This system is derived embryologically from the mesenchyme and is composed of soft and hard connective tissues. These tissues have evolved to serve two basic functions: structural integrity and stable mobility. The tissues are composite materials made up of cells lying within the extracellular matrix they produce.

Conditions in Orthopedic Physical Therapy

Orthopedic physical therapy focuses on treating conditions affecting the musculoskeletal system, which is made up of your joints, muscles, bones, ligaments, and tendons. Orthopedic injuries and conditions may include:

- Fractures
- Muscle strains
- Ligament sprains
- Post-operative conditions
- Tendonitis
- Bursitis

An injury to a bone, joint, tendon, ligament, or muscle may cause pain, limited functional mobility, and loss of strength or range of motion. These impairments may prevent you from enjoying your normal work or recreational activities. The focus of orthopedic physical therapy is to help your injury heal properly and improve your strength, range of motion, and overall functional mobility.

After surgery, you may have specific limitations that your surgeon wants you to adhere to. Your orthopedic physical therapist can help guide you through your post-operative rehab program to get you back to your normal lifestyle quickly and safely.

Any condition that causes pain or limited functional mobility as a result of an injury to bony or soft tissue structures in your body may benefit from the skilled services of orthopedic physical therapy.

Tools of the Trade

Your orthopedic physical therapist uses specific tools to help you during your rehab. These may include:

- Therapeutic modalities like heat, ice, ultrasound, or electrical stimulation
- Assistive devices, such as walkers or canes
- Orthotics and prosthetics
- Exercise tools and equipment
- Evaluation and assessment tools
- Mobilization or soft tissue massage instruments

While your PT may use various instruments and tools to help you move better and get better, exercise is often your main tool to help you recover fully and prevent future orthopedic problems. Exercises in orthopedic physical therapy often involve:

- Strengthening exercises
- Stretching and flexibility exercises
- Exercises to improve range of motion
- Balance exercises
- Functional mobility exercises
- Endurance exercises
- Plyometric and jumping-type exercises

Your orthopedic physical therapist can teach you the right exercises for your specific condition that can help you regain your normal mobility. The exercises you do in an orthopedic physical therapy may also be done at home as part of a home exercise program.

How to Become an Orthopedic Physical Therapist

Step 1: Attain a Bachelor's Degree

A bachelor's degree in biology or related field is the first step to becoming an orthopedic physical therapist. Graduate degree programs in physical therapy have certain prerequisites that must be met for admission into a doctoral degree program. Generally, the bachelor's degree courses should include minimum required courses in anatomy, biology, chemistry or biochemistry, physics, physiology, and calculus. These courses must include labs, and the student must maintain a minimum required grade point average. Some programs also require the student to have participated in minimal clinical observation.

Step 2: Attain a Graduate Degree

All states require physical therapists to have doctoral degrees. It takes three years of full time attendance after a bachelor's degree to graduate from a doctoral degree program in physical therapy. Courses generally include fitness and exercise, prosthetic and orthotic interventions, cardiovascular/pulmonary systems, musculoskeletal system, lifespan development, and treatment modalities. There are also annual clinical internship requirements where students shadow doctors and participate in physical therapy in clinical settings.

In order to be successful in a physical therapy career, verify the accreditation of the doctoral program. Make sure a Doctor of Physical Therapy program is accredited by Commission on Accreditation in Physical Therapy Education (CAPTE). Most states won't issue a physical therapy license to graduates of non-accredited physical therapy programs.

Also, make sure to follow all application requirements. Many schools require applicants to submit their transcripts, letters of reference, personal essays, and other admission documentation through the Physical Therapy Centralized Application Service (or the PTCAS). PTCAS compiles the required information and provides it to the schools to which the applicant applies.

Find Schools that Offer these Popular Programs

- Art Therapist
- Dance Therapist
- Kinesiotherapist
- Music Therapist
- Occupational Therapy
- Physical Therapy
- Prosthetics and Orthotics
- Rehabilitation Technologies
- Therapeutic Recreation
- Vocational Rehabilitation Counselor

Step 3: License and Requirements

After completing a physical therapy program, physical therapists must be licensed by the state in which they practice. The licensing process includes filing an application with proof of attendance at an accredited program, paying a filing fee, and passing a written and/or oral examination. Good moral character is also a common state licensing requirement for which applicants must qualify. Many state boards also reserve the right to impose additional licensing requirements as the situation or case demands before granting a license to practice.

In addition to this, most states have continuing competency requirements that physical therapists must fulfill to maintain their licenses. These requirements vary from state to state. There are national organizations, such as the Federation of State Boards of Physical Therapy, that provide continuing competence resources for physical therapists that conform to each state's requirements.

Make sure filing deadlines are met. Physical therapists must be sure to satisfy the continuing competency requirements and file their applications for license renewal by the deadline required by the state of employment. Failure to meet these deadlines can result in therapists being suspended for non-compliance with filing requirements.

Step 4: Orthopedic Certification

The American Board of Physical Therapy Specialties (ABPTS) provides board certification in orthopedic physical therapy. Applicants are required to be licensed as physical therapists and to have accumulated a minimum of 2,000 hours of direct patient care as orthopedic physical therapists within the prior three years. Applicants must also submit proof of participation in a research project directly related to orthopedic physical therapy within the previous ten years. They must also pass a written examination administered by the certifying board. Upon successful completion of the requirements, physical therapists will be issued board certification in orthopedic physical therapy.

Licensed physical therapists may consider gaining specialized training in orthopedics through a professional certificate program or residency, both of which can help physical therapists fulfill board certification requirements. Programs, such as a musculoskeletal physical therapy certificate program, can provide therapists with advanced knowledge in areas like neuromuscular tissues, motor control, the lumbar spine, and upper extremities. Depending on the school, classes taken in a professional orthopedic certificate program may be part of the overall requirements for a residency.

So a physical therapist working with patients and devising treatment plans and who has earned a doctorate degree in physical therapy from an accredited program, which is three years of study after earning a bachelor's degree, can, as a licensed physical therapist, work to complete the requirements for an orthopedic physical therapist certificate.

Geriatric Physical Therapy

Geriatric physical therapy was defined as a medical specialty in 1989 and covers a broad area of concerns regarding people as they continue the process of aging, although it commonly focuses on older adults.

Geriatric physical therapy covers a wide area of issues concerning people as they go through normal adult aging but is usually focused on the older adult. There are many conditions that affect many people as they grow older and include but are not limited to the following: arthritis, osteoporosis, cancer, Alzheimer's disease, hip and joint replacement, balance disorders, incontinence, etc. Geriatric physical therapists specialize in providing therapy for such conditions in older adults.

Among the conditions that may be treated through the use of geriatric physical therapy are osteoporosis, arthritis, alzheimer's disease, cancer, joint replacement, hip replacement, and more. The form of therapy is used in order to restore mobility, increase fitness levels, reduce pain, and to provide additional benefits.

Geriatric physical therapy is a proven means for older adults from every level of physical ability to improve their balance and strength, build their confidence, and remain active. A number of people are familiar with physical therapy as a form of treatment to pursue after an accident, or in relation to a condition such as a stroke. Physical therapy is useful for many additional reasons, such as improving balance, strength, mobility, and overall fitness. All of these are factors which older adults may benefit from, contributing to their physical abilities and helping to maintain their independence for longer periods of time. Physical therapy can also help older adults to avoid falls, something that is crucial to this population.

Falling is one of the greatest risks older adults face, often leading to things such as hip fractures which then lead to a downward health spiral. In fact, falling is such an issue among older adults that the Center for Disease Control and Prevention has reported that one-third of all people over the age of sixty-five fall every year, making falls the leading cause of injury among people from this age group. Hundreds of thousands of older adults experience falls and resulting hip fractures every year, with resulting hospitalizations. Most of the people who experience a hip fracture stay in the hospital for a minimum of one week, with approximately twenty-percent dying within a year due to the injury. Unfortunately, a number of the remaining eighty-percent do not return to their previous level of functioning. Physical therapy can help older adults to remain both strong and independent, as well as productive.

Forms of Geriatric Physical Therapy

Exercise: Exercise is defined as any form of physical activity that is beyond what the person does while performing their daily tasks. Exercise is something that is designed to both maintain and improve a person's coordination, muscle strength, flexibility and physical endurance, as well as their balance. It is meant to increase their mobility and lessen their chance of injury through falling. Exercise in relation to geriatric therapy might include activities such as stretching, walking, weight lifting, aquatic therapy, and specific exercises that are geared towards a particular injury or limitation. A physical therapist works with the person, teaching them to exercise on their own, so they may continue their exercise program at home.

Manual Therapy: Manual therapy is applied with the goals of improving the person's circulation and restoring mobility they may have lost due to an injury or lack of use. This form of therapy is also used to reduce pain. Manual therapy can include manipulation of the person's joints and muscles, as well as massage.

Education: Education is important to the success and effectiveness of geriatric physical therapy. People are taught ways of performing daily tasks safely. Physical therapists also teach people how to use assistive devices, as well as how to protect themselves from further injury. Older adults can utilize physical therapy as a means for regaining their independence. Physical therapy can help seniors to feel better, as well as to enjoy a higher quality of life.

Physical Therapists

Physical therapists provide people with a variety of services. They work with people individually, evaluating their physical capabilities and designing specific programs of exercise, education and wellness for them. Physical therapists also work with other health care providers to coordinate the person's care.

Physical therapists must have completed their coursework in the biological, medical, psychological and physical sciences. They must have graduated from an accredited education program, and have completed a bachelors, masters, or doctoral degree with specialty clinical experience in physical therapy. Many physical therapists choose to seek additional expertise in clinical specialties, although every physical therapist must meet licensure requirements in their state.

The potential for age-related bodily changes to be misunderstood can lead to limitations of daily activities. The usual process of aging does not need to result in pain, or decreased physical mobility. A physical therapist can be a source of information for understanding changes in the body, they can offer assistance for regaining lost abilities, or for development of new ones. A physical therapist can work with older adults to help them understand the physiological and anatomical changes that occur with the aging process.

Physical therapists evaluate and develop specifically designed, therapeutic exercise programs. Physical therapy intervention can prevent life-long disability, restoring the person's level of functioning to its highest level. A physical therapist uses things such as treatments with modalities, exercises, educational information, and screening programs to accomplish a number of goals with the person they are working with, such as:

- Reduce pain.
- Improve sensation, joint proprioception.
- Increase overall fitness through exercise programs.
- Suggest assistive devices to promote independence.
- Recommend adaptations to make the person's home accessible and safe.
- Prevent further decline in functional abilities through education, energy conservation techniques, joint protection.
- Increase, restore or maintain range of motion, physical strength, flexibility, coordination, balance and endurance.
- Teach positioning, transfers, and walking skills to promote maximum function and independence within the person's capability.

There are various common conditions that can be effectively treated through physical therapy. Among the specific diseases and conditions that might affect older adults which can be improved with physical therapy are arthritis, osteoarthritis, stroke, Parkinson's disease, cancer, amputations, urinary and fecal incontinence, and cardiac and pulmonary diseases. Conditions such as Alzheimer's disease, dementia's, coordination and balance disorders, joint replacements, hip fractures, functional limitations related to mobility, orthopedic or sports injuries can also be improved through geriatric physical therapy.

How to Become a Geriatric Physical Therapist

Required Education

A master's degree or doctorate is usually required for a geriatric physical therapy position. Most states also have unique certification criteria that must be met on top of the educational requirements. A master degree or doctorate program can take 2-4 years to complete after a bachelor's degree is awarded. Students interested in becoming geriatric physical therapists take classes in human growth and development, anatomy, therapeutic techniques, and psychology.

Skills Needed

Geriatric physical therapists need to have excellent communication and motivational skills and must be physically fit. They should also be organized and need to be able to administer and understand diagnostic tests. Patience and sympathy for their clients' conditions are also needed.

Career and Economic Outlook

The increased number of elderly people in the U.S. has led to well above average job growth projections for geriatric physical therapists. As more people enter retirement and old age, the number of available jobs among all physical therapists, including geriatric physical therapists, is projected to grow by 34% from 2014 to 2024, according to the U.S. Bureau of Labor Statistics (BLS). The median annual salary among all physical therapists was reported as $84,020 by the BLS in May 2015.

Neurological Physical Therapy

The types of neurological disabilities approached by this form of physical therapy might include ALS, alzheimer's disease, cerebral palsy, Parkinson's disease, multiple sclerosis, stroke, or spinal cord injuries. Common types of impairments associated with neurologic conditions can include balance, vision, ambulation, movement, activities of daily living, speech, or loss of functional independence.

Neurological Reparative Therapy (NRT) is a new model of treatment synthesized from a compilation of literature and research on how to better the lives of individuals who suffer from a wide range of mental, emotional, and behavioral disturbances - particularly children and adolescents.

Physical therapy is very important for people who have previously experienced, or currently have a neurological disease or injury. A person's spinal cord and brain control both their sensations and their movement. An injury to a person's brain or spinal cord may cause death of cells which control specific movements and sensations, leading to loss of function. Physical therapy can help to prevent loss of function, helping a person to remain able to perform certain activities. Should a person decide to pursue decreased activity instead, they may also experience additional health problems that can include lung or heart problems, decreased independence, diabetes, and an overall reduction in their quality of life.

Following an injury there is an amount of time during which a person's cells that remain uninjured in their brain and spinal cord retain the ability to learn how to control the functions that have been lost. Physical therapists have the knowledge necessary in relation to human movement to teach people how to move correctly again. They are able to assist people in regaining some to most of the functions they have lost due to an injury. Many people can learn to live independently once again through physical therapy.

Neurological disorders affect a person's nervous system and can happen in people from all age groups. Neurological physical therapists work with people who experience neurological conditions that can include:

- Stroke
- Sciatica
- Neuropathy
- Impingement
- Fibromyalgia
- Radiculopathy
- Cerebral Palsy
- Herniated discs
- Spinal Cord Injury
- Multiple Sclerosis
- Parkinson's Disease
- Traumatic Brain Injury

Neurological physical therapists work with people to alleviate pain, improve the person's balance and coordination, and help to restore their range of movement and motion.

Neurological Physical Therapists

Neurological physical therapists are medical professionals who work in their field of therapy after receiving years of education and a license to practice. Disciplines of neurological physical therapy are also diverse and multifaceted, ranging from orthodontic to geriatric. Certified and professionally skilled therapists are registered with the American Physical Therapy Association and have undergone examination before being accepted into the board.

There are different areas of specialization within the field of neurological physical therapy.

While this may be well known among people in the physical therapy profession, it is many times overlooked by people in the general public. There are a number of books that describe the most common areas of specialization within physical therapy that people can read, as well as information right here at Disabled-World.com. You can read and found out about different areas of specialization related to physical therapy that are most appropriate to you or your family member.

One of the most complex types of physical therapy involves neurological physical therapy which, if applied appropriately, helps to ensure that the person's nerve cells and motor functions work as they should. Neurological physical therapy can effectively help to to reduce motor defects that impair the working of a person's nerve cells. Physical therapists who work in this area of specialization assist people to improve areas related to neurological dysfunction.

Physical therapy in general is a branch of rehabilitative medicine that is aimed at assisting people to recover, maintain, or improve their physical abilities. Physical therapists as a whole work with people whose movements may be impaired by disease, disability, aging, sports injuries, or environmental factors. Physical therapy may used in the treatment of any disease, pain, or injury.

The term, 'habilitation', means making a person fit, or capable of doing something. Therefore, 'rehabilitation' means making a person fit or capable of doing something they could not longer properly do, or perform at all, yet used to be able to do. In other words, rehabilitation means restoring a person's ability or abilities.

Physical therapy is a form of clinical health science, not a form of alternative therapy. Physical therapists study medical science subjects to include neuroscience, anatomy, and physiology with the goals of acquiring the health education required for the diagnosis, prevention, treatment and rehabilitation of people who experience physical problems. Physical therapists work in general practice, hospitals, as well as in their respective communities. They are also required to be fully-qualified and registered by law.

Physical therapists must become registered. They must have graduated with a university degree in physical therapy, or a health science university degree that included physical therapy courses. Qualified physical therapists are experts in the examination and treatment of neuromuscular, cardio-thoracic and musculoskeletal conditions. They are able to focus on problems and conditions that undermine a person's abilities to move and function effectively.

How to Become a Neurological Physical Therapist

The journey to become a specialist in the field of neurological physical therapy is a long and difficult one, but the rewards at the end of it are vast. A therapist in this field is one who can evaluate and treat those who suffer from diseases or injuries that affect their nervous systems. The scope of this type of work is actually huge, as everyday people struggle with difficulties that affect their bodies and their minds. Some of the problems people experience include:

- Injuries – a spinal or brain injury can be caused by anything from a car accident to a stroke. Even a tumor can put pressure on the brain and affect bodily functions because of it.

- Illnesses – a disease such as multiple sclerosis or Parkinson's disease can affect neurons in the brain that then affect the movement of the body. This is why in the case of Parkinson's, patients often get to the stage where they cannot move at all.

- Disabilities – someone born with a mental problem may struggle with certain movements. Also a childhood disability such as cerebral palsy can permanently damage parts of the brain, causing problems in the body that can never be cured.

- Birth defects – in some cases, a person may be born missing a limb or with some kind of physical or neurological deformity that makes it difficult for them to live a normal life. In cases such as this, the therapist will need to help them make the best of their disability and try to live a normal life.

Neurological physical therapy is thus specially tailored for those who suffer from any problems in their brain that cause problems in their body. Some of the more usual symptoms include dizziness, loss of balance, difficulty picking up objects, performing simple tasks or walking, and others. The main reason that therapy is needed in these cases is not necessarily to completely cure the problem, but to assist in improving the patient's quality of life.

World of Work for a Neurological Physical Therapist

In many states, therapists in this industry are easy to find and patients do not need to be referred by a doctor. Once you have done your training in this field, you will need to register with the APTA or American Physical Therapy Association, who offer a service that allows consumers to find therapists when they are in need. It is also vital that you have a website and in some cases, therapists who have qualified band together and start a practice together. This gives them a lot more capital to work with in the short term to get more clients in the long term.

Once you start working in this field, you will be doing a lot of specialized work with those who have problems with movement. Since the central nervous system controls their whole body, they will not be able to perform certain functions without this help. In some cases, they won't even be able to feel certain sensations, and may need the therapy to assist in restoring feeling.

Decreased movement and lack of sensation also lead to other health problems, and this becomes a catch-22 situation. A good neurological physical therapy specialist will know how to assist patients in feeling sensations and moving, and will be able to improve the quality of their lives by giving them exercises and helping them work past mental and physical blocks. In the case of those who are learning to use prosthetic limbs, this can literally change their lives entirely.

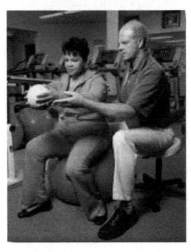

If you decide to pursue this field, you will have to be able to perform the following functions:

- Reinstate range of motion – for a number of patients, especially those affected by injury due to a sudden accident, the loss of range of motion is a big problem. They need neurological physical therapy to help them restore the amount of use they got from their limbs, especially arms and legs.

- Assist in improving strength of muscles and movement – this is a part of the therapy that will take time, since building up strength in a limb that is not being used is a difficult process. This could include going through a range of exercises to strengthen muscles and thus support the bones and joints in the body.

- Stabilizing the core – the core is such an important part of the body since it supports the spine and assists in controlling all the other parts of the body. This is why, especially when it comes to spinal injuries, it is vital to strengthen the core.

- Improving motor control – this is very important especially in terms of fine motor control. For many people who do not have control simple tasks such as using a fork and using a pen become impossible. Even larger functions such as brushing hair and picking up objects become too difficult and the quality of life is negatively affected. This is why the physical neurological therapy is needed.

- Spine realignment – spine or posture realignment is a simple procedure that sees patients assisted with straightening their spines and working unnatural curves out of their backs. This can assist in relieving muscle pain and improving the appearance, and in those with diseases such as spinal bifida or muscular dystrophy, it can greatly improve the quality of life and help in respiration, since the lungs will have more space to expand.

- Balance and gait training – it is vital if you walk to maintain balance but in some cases people cannot do this and fall easily, especially when they have been victims of a stroke. Gait training refers to the way the foot is set down and doing this correctly is also important to avoid injury. Even for runners who do not have permanent injuries, this can be particularly helpful.

- Stamina – getting the cardiovascular system used to exercise is vital for health, but many people who have been injured, especially those with brain injuries, have to retrain their bodies to not lose too much breath when they engage in cardiovascular activities, such as long walks.

- Prosthesis adaptation – for those who have lost a limb, getting used to a prosthetic limb can be very difficult, not just in terms of using the limb, but also in terms of the mental problems that come with getting used to a new limb.

- Adapting to assisting devices – for those who will be using crutches or who are confined to wheelchairs, learning to work with a device is difficult. Thus neurological physical therapy can assist with getting used to using these devices in a way that does not obstruct movement.

Neurological physical therapists work with people to alleviate pain, improve the person's balance and coordination, and help to restore their range of movement and motion. The work of a therapist in this field varies greatly depending on who they work with and on what part of the body. The specializations are as follows:

- Pediatric – as with any medical field, this is the sector that assists children who experience these difficulties. This is perhaps the easiest field to work in since children adapt more quickly than adults to certain processes.

- General – this field focuses more on those who are adults or young adults.

- Geriatric – in this field, the therapist will only deal with the elderly, and this can be very difficult because their bodies are degrading all the time, and it may be difficult to recover from injuries.

- Orthodontic – this deals more with areas of the face and jaw that need to be rehabilitated.

- Spinal – this field specializes in injuries and diseases that have affected the spine, and thus affect movement of all parts of the body.

- Podiatric/Limbs – in some cases, a person may need to retrain their limbs, especially in situations where they have been out of use, for example, when someone has broken a limb. In this case, they won't be able to use the limb for a few months, and thus will need therapy to assist them in learning to use their limbs again.

As with so many medical fields of specialization, there are many variations of neurological physical therapy that you can go into, if you want to. However, this means additional study and a lot more time spent in clinics and in research.

Studying to Become a Neurological Physical Therapist

If you have chosen to become a therapist, you will need to study at an accredited center that offers a program specializing in this type of therapy. For those who are already in the medical field, many universities and colleges will offer a specialized residency program that allows you to become a therapist in just a year.

For those who choose to study, they will need to take part in courses that offer all three of following skills development sessions:

- Teaching – the basics of the training should help you to understand the theory behind what a therapist does in this field. This means that those who teach the courses need to have practical experience that they can translate into education. Students need to be mentored by the teachers and take part in the experience of becoming a neurological physical therapist.

- Clinic – once you have mastered the theory behind becoming a therapist, you will need some practical experience in this field. This means learning the rules of practice including consulting, evaluating patients and treatment. You will also need to learn how to use new technology and how to evaluate the research you gain and turn it into statistics that can be used by others.

- Leadership – in a role such as this, it is vital that you understand the type of impact you will make on those around you. This means taking part in promoting wellness and in interacting with the community to ensure everyone is taking care of their health.

For those who wish to become students and complete this course, you need to have a thorough understanding of what is involved and that means lifelong study. This is a field in which you will learn from others, from experience and from your patients. It will be emotional and there will be times when you feel that you are not getting anywhere with a patient. Someone who chooses this career path needs to be tenacious and patient, while also being willing to work long hours.

However, the rewards of working in this field are also great, since you will definitely see an improvement in your patients and will know that you are making a big difference to their lives with your neurological physical therapy. This is not a field that everyone can work in, and though the money is good, the stresses of the job may be too much for some people to manage.

In many cases, people do not become therapists in this field unless they have done some form of therapy before, either as physiotherapists or working in orthopedics. This is because of the difficult nature of rehabilitating the human body. Patients who have to undergo this type of therapy often become despondent because the therapy is difficult, painful and can take a long time to take effect.

The job is physically challenging too, in that it requires the therapists to lift patients and assist them through their therapy. This means that they will need a lot of body strength themselves and may need to practice some of their own therapy techniques to see what the effect of these is on patients.

However, for those who succeed in this field, the rewards are both monetary and emotional. This can be a very difficult field to practice in, but when you see the results in the form of people walking, regaining their motor skills and improving the quality of their lives, it all becomes worth it. And as for those who think they can do this job just for the money, you are in for an unpleasant surprise. This is a job that is physically, emotionally and mentally draining and only those with a strong constitution, body and heart can succeed in it.

Cardiovascular and Pulmonary Rehabilitation

Cardiac Rehabilitation is a comprehensive program designed to prepare patients with heart disease for an active and productive lifestyle. Cardiac Rehabilitation has four components:

- Evaluation
- Monitored Exercise
- Education
- Support

Cardiac Rehabilitation is an outpatient service. The treatment of each patient is individualized to meet the specific patient needs. Patients attend Cardiac Rehabilitation three times per week for 6-12 weeks.

Evaluation

The admission process consists of a thorough medical history, an evaluation, and a six minute walk test.

Monitored Exercise

A significant component of Cardiac Rehabilitation is the closely monitored exercise program. Patients exercise three days per week using aerobic exercise equipment (treadmill, stationary bicycles, recumbent stepper, etc.) Patients are challenged to increase their tolerance to exercise through gradual increases in workloads. While exercising, patients have their heart rhythm, blood pressure and oxygen saturations monitored by trained healthcare professionals.

Education

Patients also have opportunities to attend group and individual education sessions that promote healthy lifestyle changes. Educational topics include diet/nutrition, risk factor modification, medications, stress management and the benefits of exercise.

Support

Patients work closely with highly trained professionals on an individual basis. Progress is monitored and adjusted as needed to help patients reach their optimal potential through a healthy approach.

Will my Insurance Pay for Cardiac Rehabilitation

Medicare, as well as most third party insurance companies, will cover Cardiac Rehabilitation. Patients are encouraged to contact their insurance provider prior to enrolling in the program.

Who is Eligible for Cardiac Rehabilitation

Those who have had a heart attack, open heart surgery, heart transplant, stable angina, PTCA/ stent, or valve repair/replacement are eligible for Cardiac Rehabilitation. A physician referral is required.

Pulmonary Rehabilitation is a program of education and exercise training that stresses proper care and symptom management for the patient with pulmonary disease. Pulmonary Rehabilitation is offered on an outpatient basis. Patients attend rehab sessions two days a week. Sessions include education about pulmonary disease and breathing techniques, as well as regular exercise.

Evaluation

Each Pulmonary Rehabilitation patient participates in an initial assessment. This includes a thorough evaluation of the patient's medical history, as well as a review of their current health condition. An exercise tolerance assessment and a physical evaluation are also performed at this time.

Monitored Exercise

An essential component of Pulmonary Rehabilitation is the exercise program, with an emphasis on impoving endurance through progressive training within the limits of each individual. The documented benefits of the exercise training include increased tolerance of shortness of breath, increased appetite, better physical capability, and improved quality of life.

Education

Patients have opportunities to attend group and individual education sessions that emphasize healthy lifestyles.

Support

Throughout the Pulmonary Rehabilitation program, patients benefit by working closely with highly trained and experienced healthcare professionals. Each patient's program is individualized to his or her needs.

Will my Insurance Pay for Pulmonary Rehabilitation?

Most insurance companies will cover Pulmonary Rehabilitation services.We encourage patients to check with their insurace provider prior to enrolling in the program.

Who is Eligible for Pulmonary Rehabilitation?

Patients with impairment due to lung disease (including emphysema, COPD, asthma, and more) are eligible. A physician referral is required.

Benefits of Cardiac and Pulmonary Rehab

Cardiac and pulmonary rehabilitation programs help improve health in both men and women who have experienced cardiac events or have been diagnosed with lung disease or disorders. Baylor Scott & White Heart – Plano works with you and your family members to make your transition back to daily life as smooth as possible. A cardiac or pulmonary rehabilitation program can help:

- Strengthen and condition your heart and lungs.
- Control your weight and lower your total cholesterol levels through good nutrition and physical activity.
- Understand your medications, the signs and symptoms of heart or lung disease, and when to seek medical attention.
- Increase your self-confidence.
- Lay the groundwork for the development of a healthier lifestyle.
- Reduce your symptoms and chances of experiencing another cardiac event.
- Develop breathing techniques and manage shortness of breath episodes.
- Return to work and activities of daily living more quickly.
- Develop coping, and stress reduction skills, and relaxation techniques.

How to Begin a Career in Cardiac Rehabilitation

A cardiac rehabilitative therapist helps patients improve their health after suffering a heart attack, undergoing a medical procedure or being diagnosed with heart disease. Therapists develop routines and set goals to help patients get back to a healthy cardiac state.

Rehabilitative therapists can work in an office or hospital environment, both of which are usually clean and climate-controlled. Although some may work evening or weekend hours, usually their work schedules conform to regular business hours. The U.S. Bureau of Labor Statistics reported the median annual salary for all physical therapists was nearly $80,000 in May 2012, as well as that they could expect to see a healthy increase in job opportunities - 36% - between 2012 and 2022. However, these professionals are often on their feet and must do a lot of physical lifting while helping their patients perform prescribed rehabilitative exercises, which can put them at risk for back injuries.

Find Schools that Offer these Popular Programs

- Art Therapist
- Dance Therapist
- Kinesiotherapist
- Music Therapist
- Occupational Therapy
- Physical Therapy
- Prosthetics and Orthotics
- Rehabilitation Technologies
- Therapeutic Recreation
- Vocational Rehabilitation Counselor

Career Requirements

Becoming a cardiac rehabilitative therapist requires an associate's degree and state licensure. The following table outlines the requirements to become a cardiac rehabilitative therapist, via the U.S. Bureau of Labor Statistics:

Degree Level	Associate's degree
Degree Field	Occupational therapy assistant
Licensure	Required; information can be found via each state's licensing/regulatory affairs department
Experience	Gained during externships
Key Skills	Attention to detail, physical stamina, good interpersonal skills
Technical Skills	Ability to use medical equipment to measure patients' vital signs
Salary	$79,860 (Median annual salary for physical therapists); $33,880 (Median annual salary for rehabilitation counselors)

Step 1: Complete Program Requirements

Working as a cardiac rehabilitative therapist requires students to complete a degree program in rehabilitative science, such as an Associate of Applied Science in Occupational Therapy, Rehabilitation Science or Physical Therapy. Prospective therapists can also choose to complete a 4-year program or earn a post-baccalaureate degree.

While aspiring cardiac rehabilitative therapists can take different career paths, certain core courses are standard for any degree program that students choose. These include an introduction to rehabilitative sciences, physical science, principles of rehabilitation science and human anatomy.

Step 2: Gain Hands-on Experience

Completing a degree program usually requires students to complete an internship through which they gain hands-on experience working with patients in medical facilities. Students take the knowledge they gained through the education process and apply it to real-life situations under the supervision of experienced professionals.

Step 3: Earn a License

Entering the field of cardiac rehabilitation can't be done without becoming licensed. Licensing requirements vary by state, but generally require the completion of an accredited degree program, passing a written licensing examination such as the National Board for Certification in Occupational Therapy (NBCOT) exam and taking continuing education courses to maintain the license.

Step 4: Consider Taking Continuing Education Courses

Maintaining a license to practice cardiac rehabilitation therapy may require professionals to take continuing education courses. Although not all states require professionals to continue the education process, taking further classes is recommended. As technology advances and new techniques and methods take the place of previous practices, professionals need to stay up to date with current industry standards.

Pediatric Physical Therapy

Pediatric physical therapy helps with the detection of health issues, using a number of modalities in order to treat disorders in children.

Therapists who specialize in pediatric physical therapy are trained to diagnose, treat and manage a variety of developmental, neuromuscular, congenital, skeletal, and acquired diseases and disorders in infants, children and adolescents. They focus on improving the person's balance and coordination, gross and fine motor skills, strength, endurance, as well as their cognitive and sensory processing and integration. Children with cerebral palsy, spina bifida, developmental delays, and torticollis are among the people who can benefit from pediatric physical therapy. Pediatric physical therapy promotes a child's independence, increasing their participation, motor development and function, improves their strength, enhances their learning opportunities, and eases care giving for family members.

A coordinated team of physical therapists and assistants develop a program that is specific to the child's needs and meets the family's goals. They work to optimize the child's gross motor and functional skills through various fun and innovative means. Pediatric physical therapists are able to work with children who have experienced or who have a brain injury, musculoskeletal or orthopedic disabilities, spinal cord injury, neurological disorders, or who have experienced a stroke, among other things.

Pediatric physical therapists have the goal of working with children in order to achieve their maximum potential related to functional independence. Through a process of examination, evaluation, and promotion of health and wellness, pediatric physical therapists implement a variety of interventions and supports. Pediatric physical therapists support children who range in age from infancy to adolescence, collaborating with their family members and educational, medical, developmental and rehabilitation specialists. They promote children and their participation and activity at home, in school, as well as in their community.

Family Member Participation

Parents and other family members of children who are pursuing pediatric physical therapy have a primary role in the child's development. A pediatric physical therapist works with family members and the individualized program that has been created for the child. Family members receive support via coordination of services, as well as advocacy and assistance designed to enhance the development of the child involved through things such as:

- Adapting toys for play
- Expanding mobility options
- Using equipment effectively
- Teaching safety for the home and community
- Positioning during daily routines and activities
- Providing information on the child's physical and health care needs
- Easing transitions from early childhood to school and into adult life

Starting a Child in a Pediatric Physical Therapy Program

Supporting a child who is going to pursue pediatric physical therapy, as well as family members, starts with an interview to identify the needs of the child. It continues with an examination and evaluation of the child in the context of their daily activities and routines. The evaluation might include their mobility, strength and endurance, muscle and joint function, posture and balance, cardiopulmonary status, sensory and neuromotor development, oral motor skills and feeding, and use of any form of assistive technologies. Providing pediatric physical therapy involves a collaborative process, coaching, as well as interventions in the child's natural learning environments. The learning environments involved can include preschools, child care centers, schools, job sites, or other community settings. Children and family members might also have contact with pediatric physical therapists from hospitals and clinics while receiving care for medical conditions that are related, or during episodes of acute care.

Pediatric physical therapy, and the provision of it, is required legislatively by the Individuals with Disabilities Education Act (IDEA), which includes provisions for pediatric physical therapy for children between the ages of birth and twenty-one years of age who are eligible for early prevention or special education services. Section 504 of the Rehabilitation Act requires the provision of reasonable accommodations, to include physical therapy, for people with disabilities. The Americans with Disabilities Act also protects the rights of people with disabilities.

Pediatric physical therapy uses evidence-based practices which integrate research findings, clinical expertise, as well as values by pediatric physical therapists to provide best practices. Pediatric physical therapists provide services to children that can include:

- Strengthening
- Motor learning
- Tone management
- Burn and wound care
- Movement and mobility
- Developmental activities
- Orthotics and prosthetics
- Balance and coordination
- Use of assistive technology
- Cardiopulmonary endurance
- Recreation, play, and leisure
- Safety and prevention programs
- Equipment design, fabrication, and fitting
- Adaptation of daily care activities and routines

Pediatric physical therapists specialize in helping children to develop and enhance their mobility so they can safely participate in activities in the community, at school, as well as at home. The therapists are concerned with the child's ability to participate in movement activities that can include crawling, walking, running, game playing, sports participation and additional physical interactions. Children who use adaptive equipment such as orthotics, wheelchairs or other forms of supports can benefit from having a pediatric physical therapist showing them how to navigate various environments. The therapists may use various intervention approaches such as massage, stretching, strengthening and endurance training to enhance a child's capabilities, as well as to prevent contractures and deformities.

How to Become a Pediatric Physical Therapy Practitioner

A pediatric physical therapist helps children of all ages recover from injuries and illnesses that affect their mobility. They also help patients with congenital conditions improve their physical abilities. Becoming a pediatric physical therapist requires extensive education, clinical hours, and licenses. In the United States, physical therapists are regulated by physical therapy associations and state boards. In addition to fulfilling all of the educational and licensing requirements, pediatric physical therapists must also be very patient and be prepared to work with children who may not understand why they must attend physical therapy sessions.

Part 1. Preparing yourself

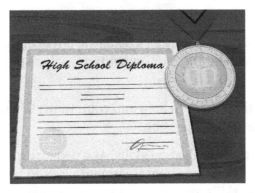

1. Graduate from high school. In order to get into an undergraduate program, you must get your high school diploma or receive your General Education Development (GED) certificate. Taking advanced science classes will help you prepare yourself for college-level studies.

- Work hard in high school and keep your GPA as high as possible to increase your chances of getting into your preferred undergraduate program.

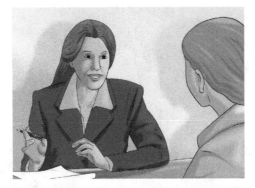

2. Gain experience. Begin exploring your interest in physical therapy by looking for after school

jobs or volunteer opportunities that will give you some experience in the field, even if you are just answering the phone.

- It might also be helpful to gain some experience working with children. Consider looking for opportunities at daycare facilities, after school programs, summer camps, children's hospitals, or pediatricians' offices.

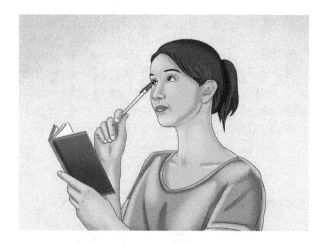

3. Assess your skills and interests. Working as a pediatric physical therapist presents many unique challenges, so it's best to think about the requirements as early as possible to make sure this career is a good fit for you.

- You must have a genuine desire to help and communicate with children in pain, which requires lots of patience and compassion.

- You must have strong communication skills. As a pediatric physical therapist, you will need to explain conditions, limitations, and treatment plans to both children and their parents. Strong communication skills are vital because communicating with children is more challenging than explaining physical therapy to adults.

- You must be prepared for physically challenging work. Pediatric physical therapists are on their feet for much of the work day and must often physically assist their patients.

Part 2. Pursuing an Education in Physical Therapy

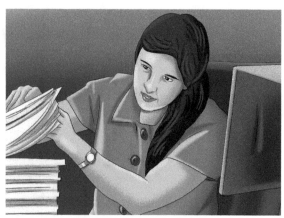

1. Get an undergraduate degree. You have many different options, so do your research to choose the best undergraduate program for you. No matter what kind of program you choose, it is important to think about the prerequisite requirements for graduate school. Consider contacting graduate schools you are interested in applying to in the future to find out what undergraduate courses are required for admission. Common prerequisite requirements include physics, psychology, and a variety of science classes.

- One option is to major in a subject that is related to physical therapy, such as biology or physiology. There are also some programs that are specifically designed to prepare you for graduate studies in physical therapy, although you can certainly be admitted to a graduate program without this specific type of major.

- Some schools offer programs that combine undergraduate and graduate studies, allowing you to earn a bachelor's degree and a doctorate degree in physical therapy from one institution without having to reapply.

- If you would like to start working in the physical therapy field as soon as possible, you may consider pursuing an associate's degree to Become a Physical Therapist Assistant. This is a great option if you want some more experience in the field before you commit to further education, or if you want to work as a physical therapy assistant while pursuing your more advanced degrees.

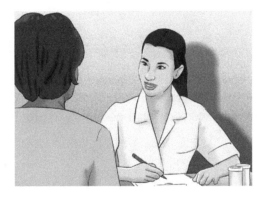

2. Apply for physical therapy internships. Many physical therapy clinics hire aspiring physical therapists to work in the office or assist with the practice. This clinical experience will give you a chance to experience what it is really like to work in a physical therapy practice, and it will add to your resume.

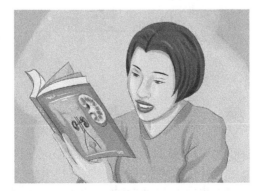

3. Attend a physical therapy graduate program. You will need to choose a doctoral program that

is accredited by the Commission on Accreditation in Physical Therapy Education (CAPTE). These Doctoral of Physical Therapy (DPT) programs generally take about three years to complete and provide you with in-depth knowledge on subjects such as anatomy and pharmacology. You will also have the opportunity to focus your studies on pediatric physical therapy.

- Prepare for graduate school by taking the GRE while you are an undergraduate. These programs are competitive, so strong grades and test scores are important.

- Master's degree programs are no longer available for new students wishing to become physical therapists, although they were an option in the recent past.

- You may be required to do an internship program as part of your DPT.

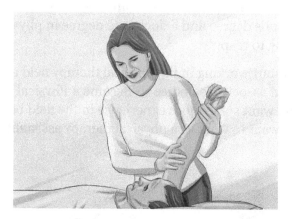

4. Complete a residency program. You will be required to complete approximately 1,500 hours' worth of clinical practice in the specialization of your choice. Residencies are usually completed at university medical centers, and will give you the opportunity to practice physical therapy under the supervision of a certified physical therapist.

Part 3. Getting Licensed and Starting your Career

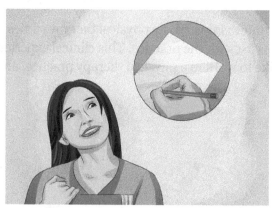

1. Get licensed in your state. You will need to take the National Physical Therapy Exam (NPTE), which assesses your knowledge and abilities in the field of physical therapy. Each state has its own requirements for issuing licenses to physical therapists, so check with your state to find out if there are additional exams you need to take.

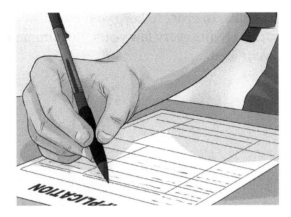

2. Apply for certification with the American Board of Physical Therapy Specialties (ABPTS). This board requires that you complete 2,000 clinical practice hours in your specialty or an approved residency program. They also administer a test for certification that includes questions related to your specialty. Upon completion of this test, you will be certified as a specialist in pediatric physical therapy.

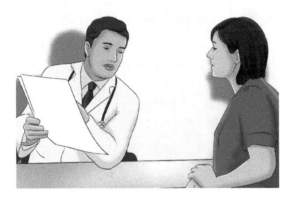

3. Start looking for your first job. Apply for jobs with hospitals, clinics, or physical therapy practices. Few pediatric physical therapists can start their own practice right away because they have a smaller pool of patients to draw from. A pediatric hospital or organization may be a great place to look for your first position.

- You can also choose to begin working as a physical therapist after you receive your license, but before you obtain certification from the ABPTS.

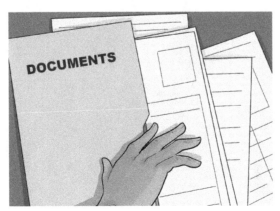

4. Take continuing education credits. In order to keep your certification and license, you will have to complete continuing education credits every few years. Requirements vary by state, so be sure to check the requirements in your area.

CHAPTER 3

Physical Therapy Treatments

Physical therapy services can be provided as primary care treatment along with other medical services. This chapter has been carefully written to provide an easy understanding of the varied physical therapy treatments for the management of muscular dystrophy, arthritis, osteoporosis and for recovery from surgery, stroke, sports injuries, back pain, etc.

How to do Physical Therapy Exercises for the Feet

The human foot is made of 26 bones and approximately 100 muscles, tendons, and ligaments. It is also the part of the body that bears the most weight, so it is not uncommon to suffer from foot pain or diagnosed foot problems at some point in your life. Painful foot problems include bunions, pronation, fallen arches, hammertoes, plantar fasciitis and tight, cramping muscles. You can fix many of these problems by performing foot exercises to stretch the muscles and reduce tension.

Method 1. Performing Foot Strengthening Exercises

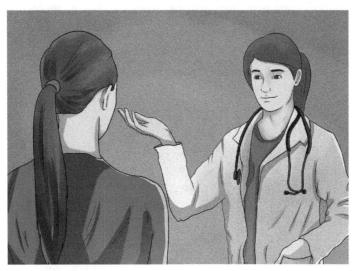

1. Seek advice. If you are experiencing foot or ankle pain, you need to get advice from your doctor or podiatrist. If the pain does not go away, even with rest, ice, and elevation, you may have a fracture. This is even more likely if there is swelling, bruising, or discoloration. You will need to seek medical treatment and get an X-ray to confirm or rule out this possibility.

- If you do have a fracture or other injury such as the ones mentioned above, ask your doctor if there are prescribed physical therapy exercises that you can do.

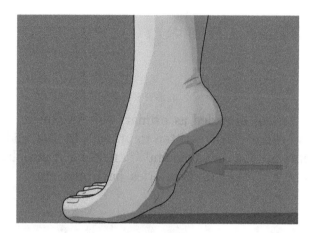

2. Try toe lifts. Sit in a chair with your feet flat on the floor. Lift your big toe up off the floor slightly while leaving the other four down. Practice this to the point where you can eventually raise up all five toes, one at the time, beginning with the big toe and ending with the fifth toe. Then practice lowering each toe one at a time, beginning with the fifth toe and ending with the big toe. Do two sets of 15.

- If you find this difficult at first, just raise your big toe up and down until you get the hang of it. Move slowly through your toes, working up to where you can do all five.

- This exercise is meant to strengthen the extenders, one of the groups of muscles which move the toes up and down. Strong extenders and flexors can help greatly with gait and balance and thus help prevent foot injuries from accidents, according to the Summit Medical Group.

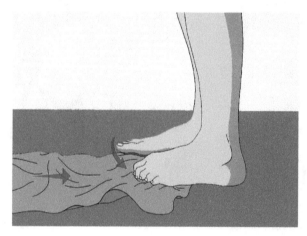

3. Do toe curls. Place a towel on the ground under your right foot. Stretch your toes out and pull them back in to grip the material with your toes. Lift the cloth one to two inches off the ground and hold for five seconds. Lower it to the ground. Repeat five times. Then repeat on the left side.

- Relax your muscles between each grip.

- Work up to holding the grip for 10 seconds at a time.

- Toe curls focus primarily on strengthening the toe flexors.

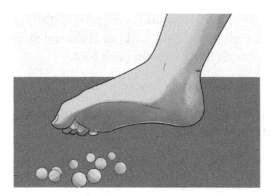

4. Pick up marbles. Place 20 marbles and a small bowl on the ground. Sit on the couch or in a chair, relaxed all the way back. With one foot, pick up one marble at a time and place it in the bowl. Then empty the marbles out and do the same thing with your other foot. This exercise will strengthen the intrinsic and extrinsic muscles in the feet. It is also helpful for plantar fasciitis but also for injuries like turf toe, a term use for injury to the great toe caused by hyperextension.

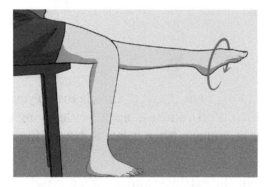

5. Write the alphabet. Sit on the couch, relaxed against the back. Extend one of your legs and raise one foot several inches off the ground. Trace the alphabet in the air using your big toe as a "pencil." Then switch legs and do the same with the opposite big toe. This exercise helps to strengthen the extensor and flexor muscles in the foot.

- It can also help with plantar fasciitis and turf toe, among other foot conditions. It is especially effective in ankle rehabilitation.

- Keep your movements small. Just use your ankle, foot, and toe.

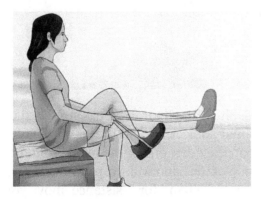

6. Do a toe extension. Wrap a rubber band around the middle of all five of your toes on your right

foot. It should have medium resistance so that it will give slightly. Stretch all of your toes apart. This will cause the band to stretch as far as it will go. Hold the stretch for five seconds and then relax your toes. Perform this stretch five times on each foot.

- Make sure to relax for approximately five seconds.

- This strengthens the extrinsic and intrinsic muscles of the foot and is used in the treatment of both plantar fasciitis and turf toe.

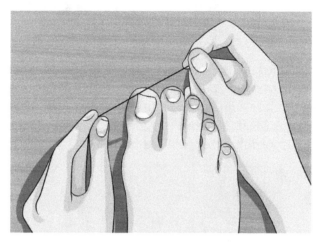

7. Try a big toe pull. Loop the rubber band between the big toe on your right foot and the big toe on your left. Place your feet together. Pull your toes apart while trying to keep your ankles together. Stretch the rubber band as far as you can, then relax. Relax for five seconds in between stretches and repeat five times.

- This exercise strengthens the extrinsic and intrinsic muscles in the feet.

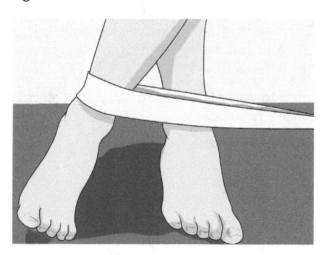

8. Do resistant ankle inversion. Sit on the floor with legs stretched out in front of you. Attach one end of a therapy band to a stationary object, such as the leg of a heavy table. The table should be beside you, down at your feet. Loop the other end of the band around the ball of your foot. The table leg will be off to the side. The loop of the band will wrap around the ball of your foot and extend out beside you toward the table. Using the band for resistance, move your ankle away from the table, pulling against the band to stretch it out.

- Do two sets of 15.

- This exercise can help to strengthen the malleolus and tibialis muscles on either side of the ankle. It can also help prevent or treat sprains.

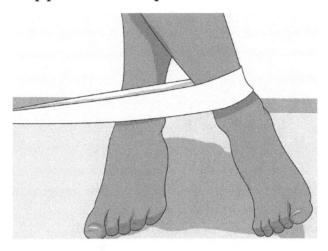

9. Perform resistant ankle eversion. This exercise is very similar to the inversion. Sit on the floor with legs stretched out in front of you. With the band in the same position as with the inversion, move the loop of the resistance band down so that it is against the arch of the foot instead of the ball. Move your foot up and out against the therapy band.

- Do two sets of 15.

- This exercise can help to strengthen the peroneal and tibialis muscles on both sides of your ankle. It can also help treat or prevent sprains.

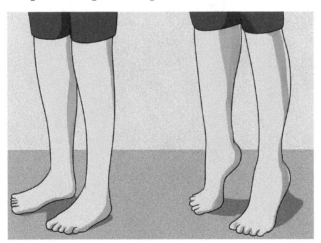

10. Do calf raises. Stand straight in front of a wall, counter, or other stable object. Place your hands gently on the wall in front of you. Raise yourself onto your toes in a calf raise exercise. From this raised-toe position, lower your feet to the ground again while keeping yourself balanced with your hands against the wall. Repeat 10 times, making sure to lower yourself slowly to the ground.

- For an extra challenge, try raising yourself on 1 foot at a time, and doing 10 reps with each foot.

Method 2. Doing Foot and Ankle Stretching Exercises

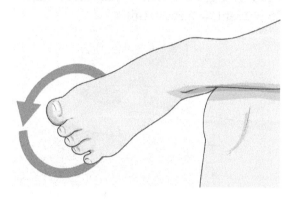

1. Test your ankle range of motion. Sit with your legs stretched straight out in front of you. Without moving legs, point your feet backward towards your body as far as they will comfortably go. Hold for 10 seconds. Then, point your toes down away from your body. Hold for 10 more seconds. Next, point toes towards the opposite foot and hold for 10 seconds. Then, point your toes away from the opposite foot and hold for 10 more seconds. Lastly, move the ankles 10 times clockwise and 10 times counterclockwise.

- This exercise was developed by the Summit Medical Group, a rehabilitation center, to help increase the range of motion or flexibility of the ankles.

- According to Summit, increased flexibility and strength in the ankle muscles, especially the tibialis muscles, can help to greatly reduce injuries such as sprains.

- Use this series as a warm-up for the remaining stretching exercises.

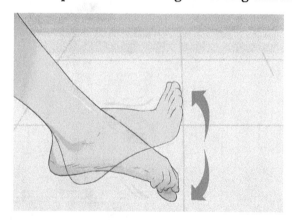

2. Do plantar flexion. This stretch is similar to the warm up, but it is a more targeted stretch. Sit against the couch with your feet straight out in front of you, so that they are perpendicular to your legs. Flex your feet back towards you as far as they will go while keeping your legs flat on the ground. Try to keep your feet extended, so your toes and heels move in a straight line. Hold for five seconds. Relax and then push your toes away from the body as far as they will go.

- Repeat 15 times, moving both feet at the same time. You can also do this exercise while you are lying down.

- To get a deeper stretch, you can use an elastic band.

- Pointing the toes away from the body helps to strengthen the muscles in the calves.

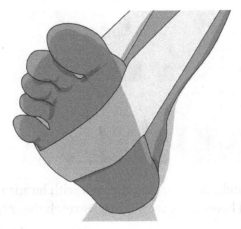

3. Try dorsiflexion. Sit in a chair and flex your right foot. Loop a large towel under your foot. Pull on the ends of the towel and pull it toward you. Stretch your toes towards you as far as you can while remaining comfortable. Hold stretch for 10 seconds and repeat 3 times with each foot.

- This stretches the muscles in the shins. Flexible shins, like calves, are important for full recovery from plantar fasciitis.

- You can also do this with a resistance band on the floor. Hook the band around a table leg. Walk away from the table and loop your foot in the band. Bring your toes toward you, pulling against the band.

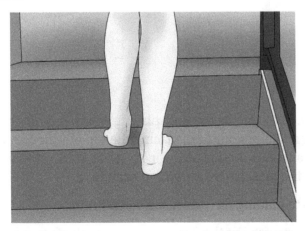

4. Do an Achilles stretch. Stand on a stair. Move until you are only standing on the stair with the balls of your feet. Hold onto the railings or wall on both sides for balance. Slowly lower your heel towards the step below you until you feel the stretching in the calf muscles. Hold this pose for 15-30 seconds, then relax. Do three reps.

- This exercise helps stretch out the muscles of the calf. Calf muscle stretching, according to the American Orthopedic Foot and Ankle Society, is integral to the treatment of plantar fasciitis. This is because excessively tight calf muscles make it more difficult to properly flex and stretch the heel. This is necessary to help recover from this painful condition.

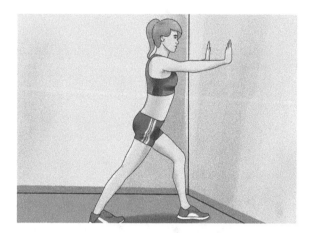

5. Perform a standing calf stretch. Stand facing the wall with hands resting on the wall for balance. Step forward with one leg and bend the knee slightly. Stretch the other leg behind you so that your heel is resting on the floor. Then, lean slowly into the wall until you feel the stretching in your calf. Hold for 15–30 seconds and do three reps.

- This exercise stretches the soleus, one of the major muscles in the calf..

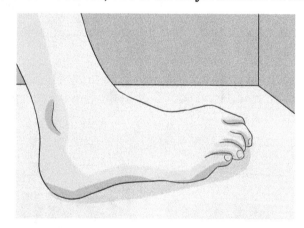

6. Stretch your toe flexors. Stand facing the wall, placing your hands on the wall for balance. Stretch your leg out behind you and point your foot, placing the top of your foot on the ground. Relax and feel the stretching in the ankle. Hold this pose for 15–30 seconds, stopping to rest for a moment if you feel any cramping in the toes. Do three reps on each foot.

- Work yourself up to holding the stance for one minute.

- This is designed to stretch out the flexors muscles in the foot, which help you move the feet in relation to the leg.

7. Roll stretch. Using a frozen water bottle, roll it back and forth with the arch of the foot from your toes to your heels. You can also use a rolling pin, a can or a tennis ball, for example, but using something cold will help reduce inflammation. You can do this either standing or sitting. This dynamic stretch is great for a long day on your feet or to help relieve stiffness or swelling.

- This exercise will strengthen the plantar fascia and other tissues that help support it, such as the Achilles tendon and calf muscles.

Method 3. Massaging your Feet

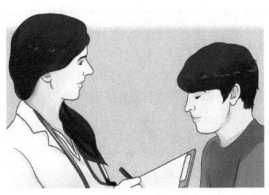

1. Know the importance of massage. Doctors and clinics such as the Sports Injuries Clinic endorse foot massage. They are relaxing, but massages also increase circulation to the feet. They also help prevent injuries such as muscle strains or sprains.

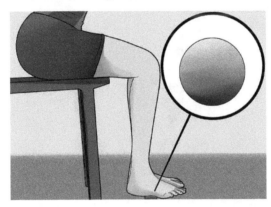

2. Perform a ball roll. Sit on a chair and place a tennis, lacrosse, or golf ball under the ball of your right foot (a tennis ball is probably the most comfortable for your foot). Roll the ball with your feet, moving the ball along the bottom of your foot from ball to heel. Continue the movement for two minutes. You should feel the massage throughout your foot.

- Try moving the ball up and down and in circles to increase the efficacy of the massage. Repeat on left foot for 2 minutes.

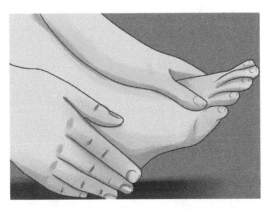

3. Give yourself a plantar fascia massage. While sitting on the chair, place your right foot on top of

your left thigh. Use your thumb to gently work circles into your arch. Run your hands up and down your foot, releasing the muscles through the whole foot. Place your fingers between your toes as if you were holding hands with your feet. Keep this position with your toes spread for 30 seconds. Massage each toe to release extra tension.

How to Treat Muscular Dystrophy with Physical Therapy

Muscular dystrophy is a genetic disorder where the body does not create enough protein to support muscle strength. There are several types of the disorder, and your diagnosis can affect the type of treatments you use. There isn't a known cure for muscular dystrophy, so prescribed treatments help to lessen symptoms, increase mobility, and slow the progression of the disease. Physical therapy is used in muscular dystrophy treatment for patients young and old. The exercises can increase muscle strength and range of motion.

Part 1. Consulting with your Doctor

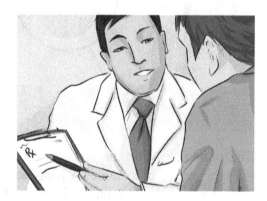

1. Create a treatment plan with your doctor. Many people suffering from this disease begin using corticosteroid medications; however, they come with risks of bone fracture. Discuss your options with your doctor at the onset of the disease, if possible.

- Your doctor will be able to advise you every step of the way and help you find the right course of treatment for your muscular dystrophy.

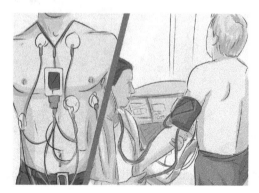

2. Stabilize your breathing and heart functions. Exercise can lead to an increase in blood pressure and shortness of breath, so make sure you undergo tests on your cardiovascular and respiratory systems before you start doing physical therapy.

- Doctors may prescribe an oxygen machine, sleep apnea device or ventilators for muscular dystrophy patients that have problems with breathing.

- In severe cases, a pacemaker may be inserted into the body to regulate the beating of the heart.

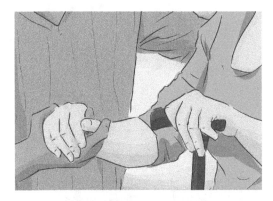

3. Request mobility aids. If you are suffering from muscle weakness, your doctor may prescribe a cane, wheelchair, or walker to reduce the risk of falling. These will help you with mobility issues around your home, and when you venture out in public.

- Your doctor may recommend that you try a full physical therapy regime first before using an aid, or they may suggest you use an aid when performing the exercises.

4. Request a prescription for your physical therapy. Using a service that is requested by your doctor and supported by your health insurance company will reduce the cost of physical therapy. Inquire about physical therapy appointment limits with your insurance company.

- Ask for recommendations of physical therapists who specialize in muscular dystrophy. People with specialized knowledge of the condition are more likely to be effective.

- Call several physical therapy offices to inquire about their experience with your specific type of muscular dystrophy.

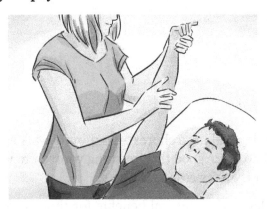

5. Begin physical therapy treatment with supervised exercise. It may take several weeks or months

before you are able to develop an at-home exercise routine. Take your time choosing a physical therapist and undergo an initial consultation.

- Choose a therapist that is recommended by your doctor (or friends), that is well qualified, that you get along with well, and that you feel is invested in your treatment.

Part 2. Practicing Low-impact Exercises

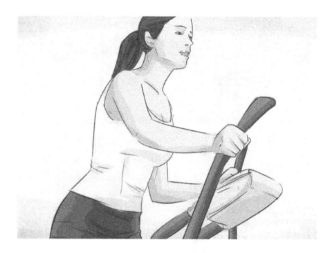

1. Begin low-impact cardiovascular exercise. Under the guidance of your physical therapist, begin regular swimming, walking on flat surfaces, and/or bike riding. Schedule exercise that is energizing, rather than tiring.

- The aim of regular exercise is to keep muscles in shape. It can also reduce weight, leaving a lower burden on joints, tendons, and muscles.

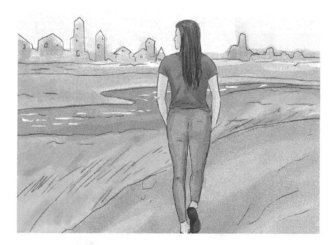

2. Walk a short distance each day. Taking a short 10-20 minute walk every day can be very beneficial for your muscles and will do more good than pushing yourself to walk an hour or more. More frequent short walks are better than fewer longer walks.

- Low-impact exercise has more physical benefits for those with muscular dystrophy than high-impact exercises that encourage cramping the next day.

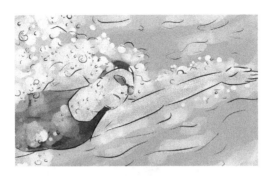

3. Go for a short swim. Try swimming laps for a short period of time (around 10-20 minutes) once every day or so. This shorter activity period will be easier on your body and will benefit you more than fewer, longer swimming sessions.

- Overworking your body with intense exercise is actually detrimental for those who have muscular dystrophy.

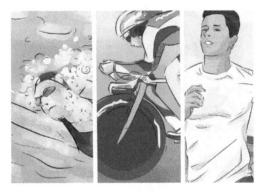

4. Try other exercises to diversify your workouts. Remember that you need to try to work out different muscles through varying exercises. Performing the same workout routine over and over will only concentrate on a specific group of muscles, while overlooking the rest.

- Focus on arms one day, then switch to legs the next. Do some low-impact aerobic exercises during one workout session, then change it up with some strength training during your next workout.

- Consider using an elliptical machine (on a low setting) or a stationary bicycle for a relatively low-impact workout.

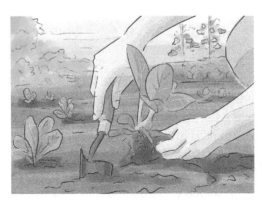

5. Work in your garden. Gardening can be a great way to include physical activity in your daily life.

It involves bending, standing, lifting, digging, and just being generally active. You'll be outdoors, moving around, and using your muscles.

- You may also get a sense of personal satisfaction at watching something grow that you worked on yourself.

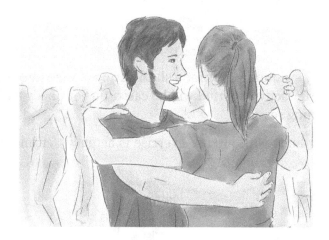

6. Take ballroom dancing classes. Ballroom dancing is another recommended method of adding more physical activity to your life. It is a low-impact activity that most people are capable of doing. It requires you to walk, move your arms and legs, and keeps you exerting energy for periods of time.

- You can also try other forms of dancing – like line dancing or square dancing.

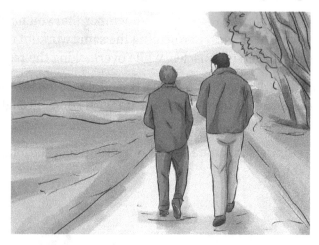

7. Participate in active recreation activities to increase happiness. Living with muscular dystrophy can take a toll on you emotionally. It's important to maintain your mental health, as well as your physical health. Including active recreational events in your life, especially those with a social aspect, may help you feel more connected and more in control of your life.

- Try going to a picnic hosted by your church or participating in a parade in your community.

- Try gentle yoga or Tai Chi, which can be done alone or in a group setting. Both offer relaxation and mindfulness aspects, which can help you cope with pain.

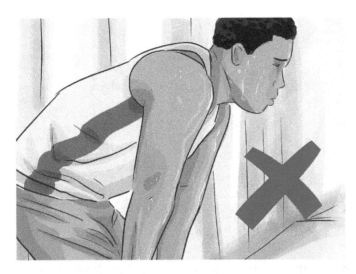

8. Avoid pushing yourself too hard. Take care while you are exercising to make sure you can handle the exertion. If you start to feel pain or discomfort, you should stop what you're doing immediately and give your body a break. Moving forward, try to switch to more low-impact activities that your body is better equipped to handle.

- Discuss any continued pain with your doctor.

Part 3. Doing Range-of-Motion Exercises

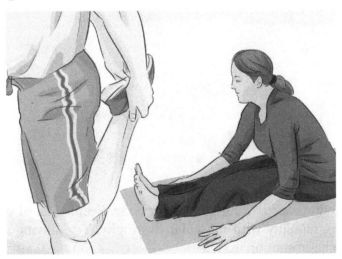

1. Develop a range-of-motion exercise routine. These prescribed exercises are tailored to your body to promote joint flexibility. Doing these exercises every day is likely to increase mobility and lessen your risk of contractures.

- These exercises should be simple enough to begin at home and do regularly. Stop the exercise immediately if it causes a severe increase in pain. You should not try to push your joints past the point where they move.

- Sometimes, doing exercises after warming up with cardiovascular activity will increase your mobility further.

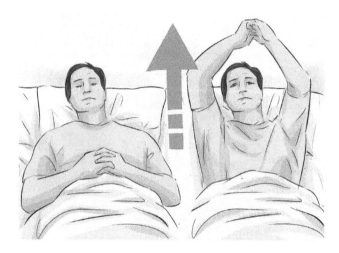

2. Do arm raises. A type of range-of-motion exercise for the shoulders involves raising your arms over your head. If you're a righty, your stronger arm will likely be your right one. To begin this exercise, you should first grasp your non-dominant arm with your dominant arm at the wrist and hold it, then raise it above your head. Hold this pose for several seconds.

- Then repeat the exercise with the dominant hand grasping the non-dominant arm.

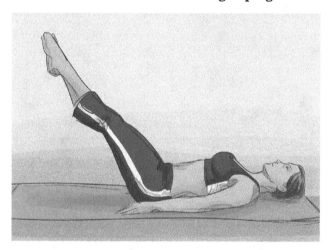

3. Practice range-of-motion exercises for your lower body. Keeping all of your joints active is important for maintaining mobility with muscular dystrophy. Try moving all of your lower body joints daily through range-of-motion exercises.

- You can lie on your back in your bed and raise one leg up in the air. Practice bending your leg at the knee and rotate the bottom half of your leg at the knee joint. Do the same with the other leg.

- Try lying on your side and lifting your leg up and down slowly.

- Even just raising your legs up and down can help with joint mobility.

- If you have trouble doing these kinds of activities on your own, you can try doing an adapted aquatic version in the swimming pool, or have someone else assist you.

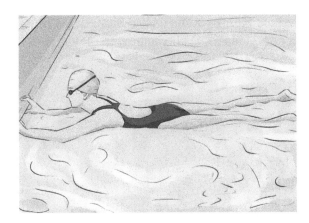

4. Try aquatic range-of-motion exercises. Research physical therapy locations that have a pool and have the therapist instruct you on how to safely exercise in the water. Performing exercises in the water gives your body an added layer of protection because the water makes your body weigh less, making the exercise even more low-impact overall.

- Try arm circles, wrist circles, bending your elbow, flexing your fingers, and moving other joints while submerged in the water.

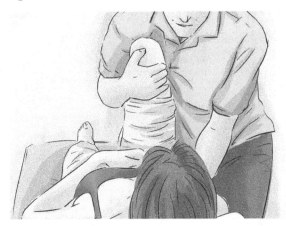

5. Return to your physical therapist to adjust your exercises. Muscular dystrophy patients must adjust their exercise routine as the condition progresses. Return every few months to assess any changes that need to be made in your plan.

- Keep your physical therapist updated about your progress, symptoms, and any impediments you might be facing. It's normal for your therapy routine to alter over time as your needs change.

How to Make Finger Weights for Hand Physical Therapy

Physical therapists sometimes recommend the use of finger weights for people dealing with arthritis or other finger joint pain. They are primarily for exercise, but wearing them while typing or playing the piano may reduce pain in some cases. Sometimes musicians use them to increase strength and speed of the fingers. This topic shows how to make them for about one percent of the cost of an expensive commercial set.

Steps

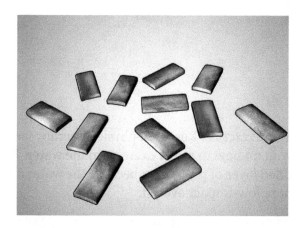

1. To make a complete set of 10, cut 50 1 inch pieces of ¼ inch (0.6 cm) copper tubing. Flatten the pieces with a hammer.

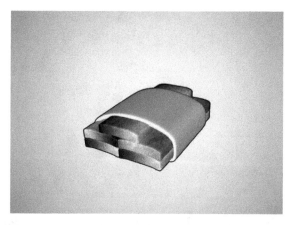

2. Lay 2 pieces on a piece of duct tape, then lay 2 more on top of those, and a 5th one on top of those. Use a total of 5 pieces. Wrap the tape around them.

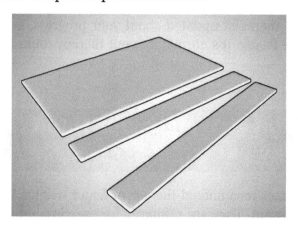

3. Cut a strip of foam craft sheet to about 1/2 inch (1.3 cm) width.

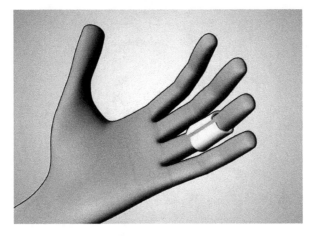

4. Wrap the strip around the finger the weight is being fitted for and cut so that the ends butt together around the finger with a medium tight fit.

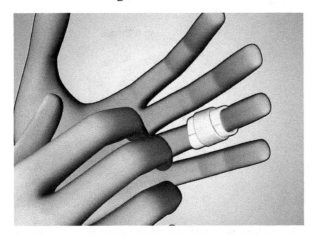

5. Tape the foam strip so that it forms a ring just fitting the finger.

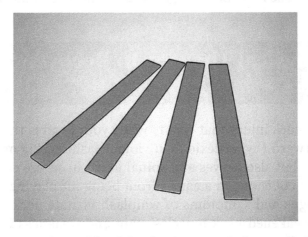

6. Cut a strip of tape about 1/3 the width of the duct tape and about 4 inches (10.2 cm) long.

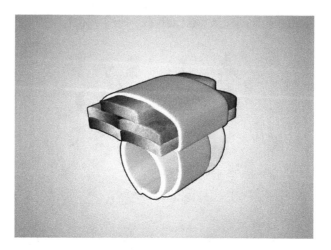

7. Use this strip to tape the packet of weights to the foam ring.

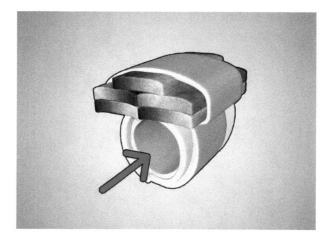

8. Optionally, tape the joint on the inside of the foam ring for greater strength so that it holds together through being taken on and off the finger. Covering the ends of the weights with tape helps prevent getting scratched. The number of weights can be adjusted to individual need.

How to use Physical Therapy to Recover from Whiplash

Whiplash is primarily a neck injury that occurs when your head is thrown backwards (hyperextension) and then forward (hyperflexion) in violent fashion. Ligaments, muscles and tendons are injured mostly, but also nerves and spinal joints in severe cases. Whiplash is often a consequence of rear-end collisions in a car or from being hit playing sports (such as football or hockey). Common signs and symptoms of whiplash include neck pain and inflammation, reduced neck motion, weakened neck muscles, pain and weakness in the shoulders / arms, headaches and dizziness. There are various forms of physical therapy that are helpful for whiplash recovery.

Part 1. Seeking Medical Attention First

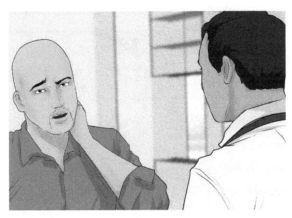

1. See your family doctor. You should seek medical attention immediately after a whiplash injury. A complicating factor is that the pain and disability of whiplash can take a day or even a week to fully manifest, but see your family physician soon after any major trauma to your head and neck in order to rule out life-threatening injuries (fractures, dislocations, internal bleeding).

- Your doctor will likely take an x-ray of your neck (cervical spine) to rule out obvious fractures or dislocations of the vertebrae or facet joints.

- If you're in severe pain and having difficulty holding your head up, then you may be given a foam neck support collar for short-term use. However, research has shown that wearing a stiff cervical collar for much more than a few days can cause neck muscles to atrophy (weaken) and prolong pain.

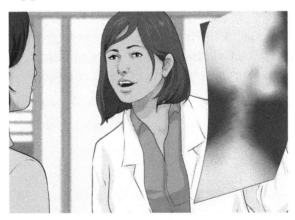

2. Make sure your neck is stable. Your family doctor is not a musculoskeletal specialist, so if your neck feels severely injured then you may need to see a specialist for a second opinion. A specialist such as an orthopedist may take more x-rays, an MRI or a CT scan of your neck / head to better understand and diagnose your whiplash injury.

- In addition to bone injuries, MRI can detect soft tissue injuries, such as spinal cord damage, herniated disks or torn ligaments.

- Before starting physical therapy your doctor(s) need to determine if your neck is structurally intact, physiologically stable and able to safely withstand stretching and exercising.

- Sharp or burning pain combined with grinding sounds with movements, shooting pains into your arms and severe dizziness are signs suggesting neck instability.

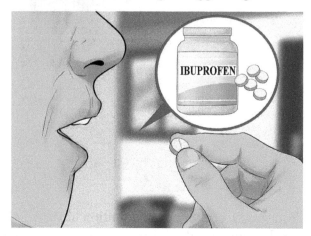

3. Control the pain and inflammation. Before you start to stretch and exercise your neck, you need to reduce the inflammation and pain. Your doctor may recommend non-steroidal anti-inflammatories (NSAIDs) such as ibuprofen or naproxen for short-term use, although if your pain is severe, you might get a prescription for something stronger — typically an opioid, such as oxycodone.

- Alternatively, you can try over-the-counter analgesics such as acetaminophen (Tylenol) or muscle relaxants (such as cyclobenzaprine) for your neck pain, but never take them concurrently with NSAIDs.

- Keep in mind that these medications can be hard on your stomach, kidneys and liver, so it's best not to use them for more than 2 weeks at a stretch.

- The application of ice is an effective treatment for essentially all acute musculoskeletal injuries, including neck pain. Cold therapy should be applied to the most tender part of your neck for 15-20 minutes every 2-3 hours in order to reduce the swelling and pain.

- Always wrap ice or frozen gel packs in a thin towel in order to prevent frostbite on your skin.

Part 2. Receiving Physiotherapy

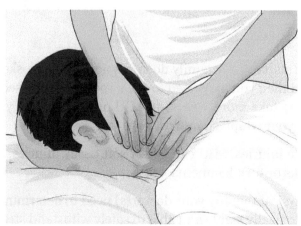

1. Get a referral to a physiotherapist. If you doctor or specialist thinks your neck is stable enough to handle the rigors of physiotherapy, then start as soon as you can. People who keep moving their necks in some capacity (even just basic stretches and mobilizations) have a better prognosis with their whiplash injuries. Your physiotherapist will assess your neck and then develop a recovery plan that includes specific and tailored stretches and strengthening exercises.

- With a referral/prescription from your doctor, physiotherapy is usually covered by private health insurance.

- For pain control, a physiotherapist can use a TENS (transcutaneous electrical nerve stimulation) unit or therapeutic ultrasound on your neck and shoulders.

- If need be, a physiotherapist can stimulate, contract and strengthen your neck and shoulder muscles with an electronic muscle stimulation device.

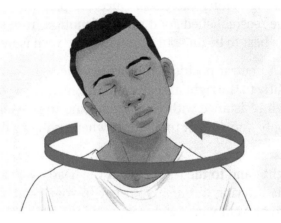

2. Start with neck stretches and mobilizations. Injured muscles and tendons quickly become tight and spasm. As soon as you can after your whiplash injury, and within pain tolerance, start stretching the muscles of the front, back and sides of your neck in order to keep them pliable. Additionally, slowly moving your neck in all directions (mobilizations) keeps the muscles flexible and prevents the spinal joints from getting too stiff. Use slow, steady movements and take deep breaths during your stretches. In general, hold stretches for about 30 seconds and repeat three to five times daily.

- Lateral neck muscle stretch: while standing, reach around your back with your right arm and grab a little above your left wrist. Gently pull on your left wrist while laterally flexing your neck in the opposite direction, such that your right ear approaches your right shoulder. Hold for 30 seconds, then do the other side.

- General neck mobilization: start with moving your head in circles, first clockwise and then counterclockwise, for about five to 10 minutes each way.

- Target the main movements of your neck: forward flexion (looking down at your toes), lateral flexion (ear towards your shoulders) and extension (looking up towards the sky). Go as far as you can in each of the four directions about 10 times daily.

- Its important to remember not to stretch into the range of motion that causes pain. If you feel pain, slightly bring your neck back until you no longer feel pain. That will be the furthest position you will need to reach for your stretching. By stretching in a pain-free range, there is less chance of irritating the injured muscle tissue, ligaments and joints.

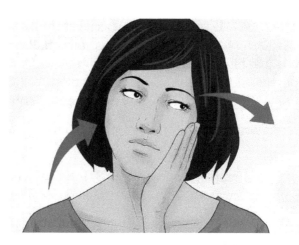

3. Progress to isometric strengthening exercises. Once the pain and inflammation in your neck has settled down and you've reestablished good range of motion from stretching, it's time to start strengthening exercises. It's best to begin your strengthening with isometric exercises.

- Keep your head in a neutral position and bring your right hand up to your right cheek. Turn your eyes slightly to the right and attempt to gently turn your head to the right, while applying just enough resistance with your right hand to prevent your head from moving. You should only apply 5 to 10% of total effort when trying to turn your neck. Repeat this five times.

- Next, place your right hand to the right side of the head. Now attempt to laterally flex the head to the right, as if trying to touch your ear to your right shoulder. Again, apply just enough resistance to prevent your head from moving (5 to 10% of total effort).

- Bring your right hand and place it on the front of your head at the forehead area. Try to bring your head forward and flexing down, but apply just enough pressure with your right hand so that your head does not move.

- Bring your right hand behind your head. Try extending your head, with just enough resistance (5 to 10%) so your head doesn't move.

- Repeat all the exercises again by using your left hand over the left side of your head. Perform this exercise three times per week.

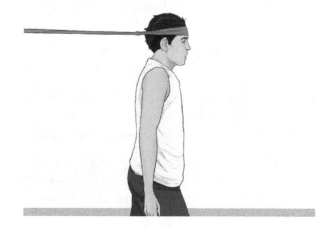

4. Try other strengthening exercises using equipment. You can strengthen your neck using exercise bands, which are usually color coded to represent different levels of tension. You may also consider newer technology, such as a multi-cervical unit.

- Tie the least resistive elastic band around your head and attach it to something stable that's at the level of your head. Walk a few steps away from it until you feel tension in the exercise band. Then do the four main neck movements (flexion, extension, right/left lateral flexion) under tension ten times each on a daily basis. After a week or so, change to a thicker exercise band with more tension.

- Advance to treatment with a multi-cervical unit. This fairly-new type of machine allows a whiplash patient to sit in a machine and attach their head to a small set of weights. Starting with light weights, you can move your neck as instructed by the physiotherapist in order to strengthen the various muscles in your neck.

Part 3. Receiving other Physical Treatments

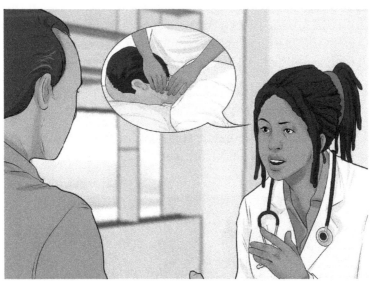

1. See a chiropractor or osteopath. Chiropractors and osteopaths are spinal specialists who focus on establishing normal motion and function of the small spinal joints that connect the vertebrae, called spinal facet joints. Manual joint manipulation, also called an adjustment, can be used to unjam or reposition facet joints that are slightly misaligned due to a whiplash injury. You can often hear a "popping" sound with a neck adjustment. Traction techniques may also help reestablish the normal curvature (lordosis) of your neck and reduce pain.

- Misaligned upper neck (cervical) facet joints greatly inhibit the ability to rotate your head and contribute to dizziness and headache symptoms.

- Although a single spinal adjustment can sometimes completely relieve your neck issue, more than likely it will take 3-5 treatments to notice significant results.

- In addition to chiropractors and osteopaths, some physiotherapists also use manual adjusting techniques for spinal and peripheral joints.

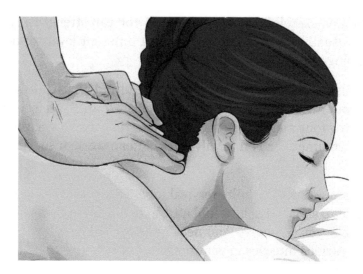

2. Get a deep tissue massage from a massage therapist. Whiplash injuries often involve significant ligament sprains and muscle / tendon strains, which leads to inflammation and spasm. A deep tissue massage is helpful because it reduces muscle spasm, combats inflammation and promotes relaxation. Start with a 30 minute neck massage, focusing also on your shoulders and muscles at the base of your skull (suboccipitals). Allow the therapist to go as deep as you can tolerate without wincing.

- Tight suboccipital muscles can trigger severe head pain called cervicogenic headaches.

- Always drink lots of water immediately following a massage in order to flush out inflammatory by-products and lactic acid from your body. Failure to do so might cause a dull headache or mild nausea.

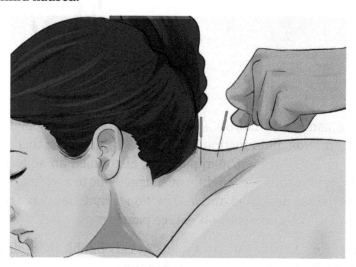

3. Consider acupuncture. Acupuncture involves sticking very thin needles into specific energy points within the skin / muscle in efforts to reduce pain and inflammation and to potentially stimulate healing. Acupuncture is not commonly recommended for whiplash recovery and should only be considered as a secondary option, but anecdotal reports suggest it can be very helpful for relieving pain and restoring mobility. It's worth a try if your budget allows for it.

- Based on the principles of traditional Chinese medicine, acupuncture reduces pain and inflammation by releasing a variety of substances including endorphins and serotonin.

- Acupuncture is practiced by a variety of health professionals including some physicians, chiropractors, physical therapists, naturopaths and massage therapists — whoever you choose should be certified by NCCAOM.

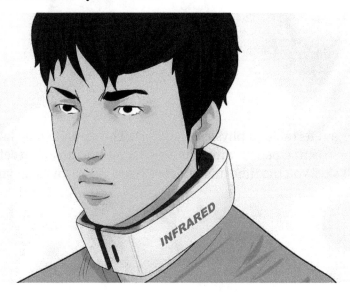

4. Consider infrared therapy. The use of low-energy light waves (infrared) is known to be able to speed up the healing of injuries, decrease pain and decrease inflammation. Use of infrared radiation (either through a hand-held device or within a special sauna) is believed to penetrate deep into the body and improve circulation because it creates heat and dilates blood vessels.

- In most cases, significant pain reduction can start within hours after the first infrared treatment.

- Pain reduction is often long lasting, weeks or even months.

- Practitioners most likely to use infrared therapy include some physical therapists, chiropractors, osteopaths and massage therapists.

How to use Physical Therapy to Recover from Surgery

Post-surgery rehabilitation or physical therapy (PT) is an important part of recovery from an injury or illness. Hospitals use physical therapists extensively, and often try to get patients moving as quickly as possible after surgery. Often, physical therapy is the only exercise you will be allowed after your surgery. Therapy strengthens your muscles after a surgery, and keeps your joints flexible. You may be asked to do therapy by yourself or work closely with a therapist as part of your rehabilitation plan.

Method 1. Planning Post-surgery PT

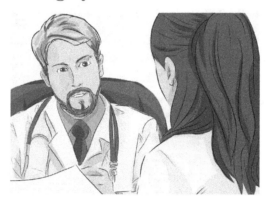

1. Ask your doctor for a referral for a physical therapist. The surgeon may know of multiple therapists with expertise on treating people with your condition. Doctors often refer patients directly to therapists, which will save you the time and effort of vetting therapists on your own.

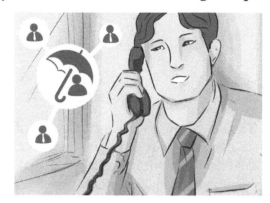

2. Find out what physical therapists are in your insurance network. Once you've been given a recommendation and/or referral from your doctor, you'll need to call your insurance company and see if your insurance covers one of these therapists. You may need to make a decision as to whether you will go to a specialized physical therapist that is not in your network or a general therapist who is covered by insurance.

- If you are interested in working with an out-of-network therapist, call them before your surgery to see what rates and discounts are available. Make the decision based on your priorities and what you can afford.

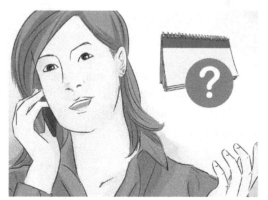

3. Find out how many therapy sessions your insurance company covers. This can be done through a quick phone call a few days before your surgery. Knowing how long your therapy sessions will be covered gives you a rough time-frame how long you can expect your recovery to take. It will also benefit your peace of mind to know how long insurance will pay for your treatment.

- The company may cover anything from a few sessions to unlimited sessions.

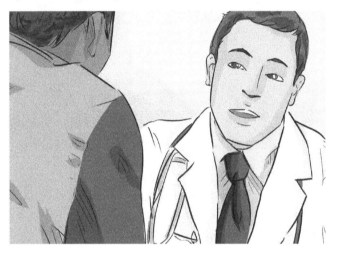

4. Discuss rehabilitation with your surgeon before surgery. Ask about what exercises you should be doing at 1 week, 1 month, and 3 months (or longer) after your surgery. Identify short-term goals, such as range of motion improvement, and long-term goals, such as a reduction in pain or an increase in overall mobility.

- Having this information ahead of time will help you stay on-track and motivated to complete your therapy.

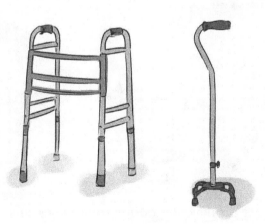

5. Buy any necessary equipment. Many surgeries require a walker, cane, resistance bands, or other exercise tools. Ask your physical therapist and doctor what you will need before you leave the hospital. You may need to purchase items from a medical-supply store located on the hospital campus.

- Your insurance company will likely cover any needed therapy supplies.

Method 2. Receiving Inpatient PT after a Major Surgery

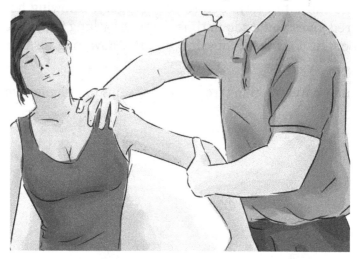

1. Have several physical therapy sessions when you are in the hospital. Physical therapists often treat new surgery patients once or twice per day in a one-on-one setting. Having therapy sessions before leaving the hospital will give you a good idea of what therapy will be like moving forward. It'll also give you a chance to ask the therapist any questions you may have about the recovery process.

- As much as you can, try to be awake, alert, and positive during these sessions.

- Your surgeon will work with your physical therapist to coordinate your care while you are in the hospital.

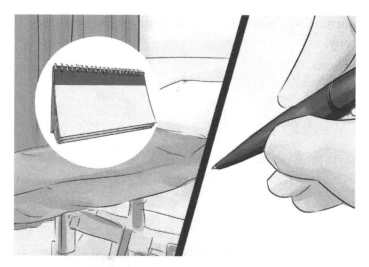

2. Ask a friend or family member to take notes during your PT sessions. This person can jot things down about exercises and recommendations the therapist makes. You may have extensive pain or be on medication that doesn't allow you to focus, and it will benefit you to have as many lucid notes as possible.

- These notes will help you develop and follow a regimen of physical therapy exercises that you can do on your own in addition to sessions with your therapist.

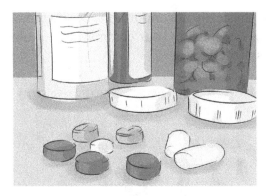

3. Take pain medication as directed by your doctor. During recovery from most major surgeries, patients are often asked to take morphine or other medications to increase their comfort and mobility. Stay on these drugs as directed and come off the pills in stages so that your body can adjust to any new pain.

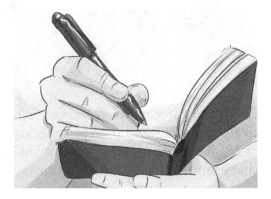

4. Keep track of the overall effect of the therapy on your body. Keep a journal of your pain, progress and questions so that you can consult the physical therapist or surgeon at post-operative visits. It's important to maintain a dialogue with your therapist so that they can alter your exercise regimen as necessary.

- For example, if you're been asked to walk on a treadmill for 45 minutes every day but feel strong pain after 20 minutes, pass this information on to your therapist.

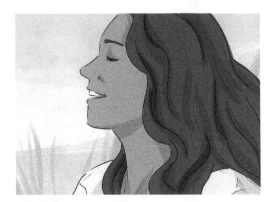

5. Stay positive as you progress through therapy. There is a mental component to physical therapy.

At time the exercises may be physically uncomfortable, or you may feel frustrated by an apparent lack of progress. Your success depends on your commitment, desire and optimism that you will recover to a healthy, mobile state.

Method 3. Doing Outpatient PT after a Minor Surgery

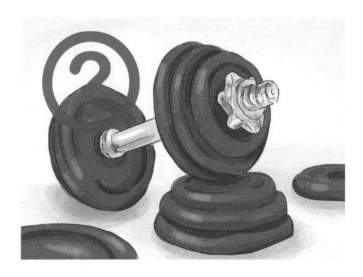

1. Ask your doctor for descriptions of required exercises. Since you'll be performing physical therapy out of the hospital, most likely with a licensed therapist that your doctor has referred you to, you'll need to have a good idea of what exercises your doctor would like you to perform with the therapist. You should know what exercises are essential to your range of motion and others that affect general mobility.

- Ask your doctor for any charts that will give you a visual on how each exercise should look. Also inquire about visual diagrams and the expected outcome of each exercise.

- For example, if you've undergone spinal surgery, you'll be asked to do exercises to strengthen your back muscles (surrounding the point of incision) and to maintain flexibility in your spine.

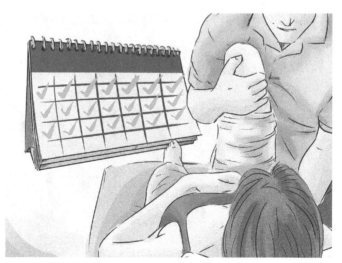

2. Make physical therapy a part of your daily routine. Physical therapy is most effective when done frequently. Just like any other type of exercise, it can be easy to forget about therapy or put it off altogether. By keeping to a daily schedule of exercise and stretches, you'll prevent scar tissue from building up around the injured area and ensure that you have a full range of motion after recovery.

- Performing your therapy daily will also decrease the slight pain or discomfort that sometimes accompanies therapy.

- For example, if your doctor has asked you to do physical therapy work on your core region following an abdominal surgery, you could do Pilates every morning before work.

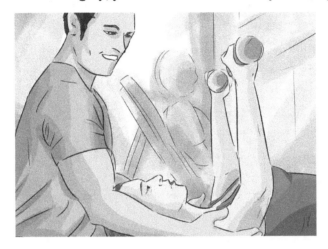

3. Regain muscle strength through physical therapy. Failing to follow through with your physical therapy regimen can have serious consequences. Doctors prescribe therapy as a way for you to build up the strength of muscle groups that were cut through (or otherwise affected) by the surgery. If you do not comply with the physical therapy, you may end up with a permanently weakened muscle group.

- The risk of permanently weakened muscles is especially high for the elderly, who often have low muscle tone prior to the surgery.

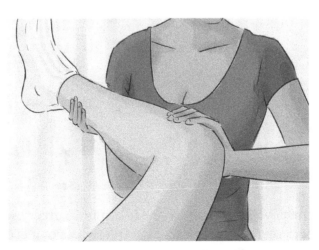

4. Maintain joint function and physical mobility with physical therapy. If you fail to complete the

regimen of physical therapy, you also run the risk of permanently losing joint flexibility. Doing the exercises as part of a physical therapy regimen will keep your joints flexible and prevent you from losing your physical mobility.

- For example, if you had surgery on your legs or knees, your doctor will prescribe you physical therapy that involves strengthening leg muscles and maintaining knee flexibility. If you don't complete the therapy, you may permanently lose the ability to walk up and down stairs.

Method 4. Performing Exercises as the Therapist Directs

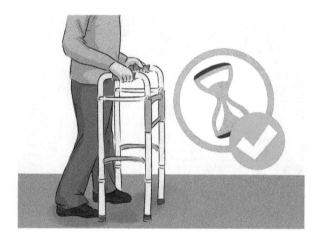

1. Follow your physical therapist's orders about the amount and duration of exercise. If these metrics or other goals are not clear to you, phone or visit your therapist to clarify what you are doing. It's always better to ask and be sure than to make mistakes in your exercise.

- Therapy is designed to maintain your flexibility and re-strengthen your muscles following surgery. However, if you perform exercises incorrectly, you risk re-injuring yourself.

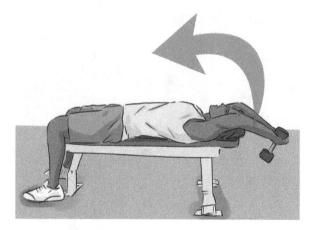

2. Work your core and stretch your back if you've had a spinal surgery. Work with your therapist to construct a core-and-back therapy routine. Plan to start with 1 or 2 exercises for your back, and perform 1-2 sets of 12-15 reps. These exercises will strengthen your core and maintain back flexibility.

- Try dumbbell pullovers. Lay on your back and hold the dumbbell over your head. Lower the weight behind you, and tense the muscles on your sides to slowly raise the weight back up over your head.

- One of the most common types of exercise for your back muscles is lat pulls with bands. Your therapist will have you hold an elastic gym band above your head and move your arms out sideways to strengthen your back and sides.

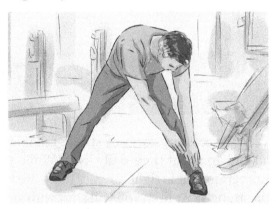

3. Maintain a good stretching regimen throughout your therapy. Stretching can both build muscle tone and improve flexibility. As your therapy progresses, your therapist will likely increase the difficulty—and duration—of the stretches you're asked to perform. Common stretches used in physical therapy include:

- Hamstring stretches, in which you'll sit with 1 leg outstretched in front of you. Reach out with your fingers and try to touch the toes of the extended foot for 15 seconds, then repeat with the other leg.

- Quad stretches, in which you'll lie on your right side, then bend back your left knee. Grasp your left ankle with your left hand, and pull towards your buttocks until you feel your quad muscle stretch. Repeat with your right leg when lying on your left side.

- Standing calf stretches, in which you'll slide your left leg 18 inches (46 cm) behind you, then lean your body weight forward over your right foot for about 15 seconds, until you feel your left calf muscle stretch. Then repeat with your right leg behind you.

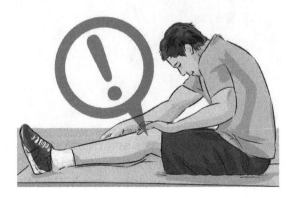

4. Stop your exercise if you feel pain while doing therapy. Therapy is designed to strengthen your

muscles and improve mobility. While it may be uncomfortable at times, it should never be painful. Stop exercising at once if you notice any bleeding from your incision, if you have excessive swelling in the area around your incision, or if you feel extreme pain.

- For example, if you've had a surgery on your knee, therapist may ask you to start doing your hamstring stretches or straight leg raise exercises (both excellent for post-knee-surgery therapy) for a longer duration of time. Stop doing the exercise and inform your therapist if you feel pain.

How to use Physical Therapy to Recover from a Stroke

Physical therapy is an effective and necessary form of stroke rehabilitation which helps people recover their ability to function and go about their daily lives. While you should work with your physical therapist to develop a program that is right for you, there are some basic movements you can learn at home to help regain strength. At first, you will start with small movements in the hospital as directed by your doctor or physical therapist. You should then start doing daily exercises to improve the use of your arms, help your balance, and increase the strength of your lower body. Make sure that you are supervised by your physical therapist or caretaker while doing physical therapy in case you hurt yourself or fall.

Method 1. Using Physical Therapy in the Hospital

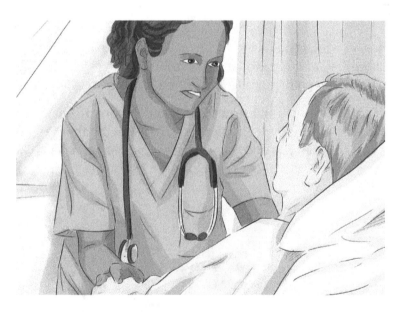

1. Meet with your physical therapist to discuss goals and treatments. Your physical therapist will tell you specifically which exercises you should be focusing on. They will take notes from your doctor and create an individualized plan. Always consult your physical therapist before adding new exercises and stretches to your regimen.

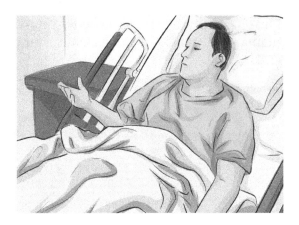

2. Start moving as soon as you can. You do not want to begin your physical therapy too soon. Most doctors will have you starting between 24 and 48 hours after the stroke. You can ask your doctor when you will be able to begin.

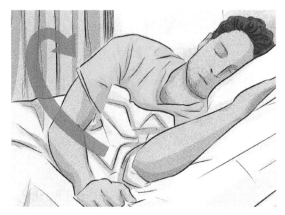

3. Change positions frequently in your hospital bed. Sit up if you are able. This will help to remind your weakened muscles how to move. You can support your body by placing a foam wedge near the small of your back.

- If you are ready, you can, with assistance, try moving from your bed to your chair. Do not try this when you are alone.

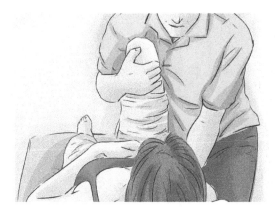

4. Work with a therapist on passive movements. Passive movements are exercises where your

therapist moves your limbs for you. You may be paralyzed after your stroke, or you may otherwise have difficulty moving. By guiding you through the movements, your physical therapist is helping you regain joint mobility.

- A common passive movement is arm rotation. Your therapist will gently move your arm in a circular motion.

- Your physical therapist may also ask you to lie down so that they can stretch and bend your legs for you.

- You should ask your therapist to teach family members or caretakers to help you with these passive movements so that they can help you even when you are discharged.

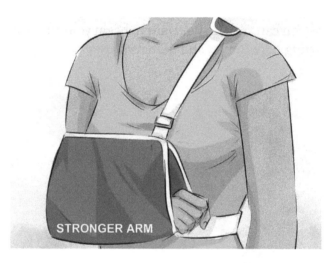

5. Wear a sling on your strong arm. If your arm was paralyzed by the stroke, wearing a sling on the healthy arm will force you to use the weak arm. This will strengthen the arm over time. Ask your physical therapist to fit you with a sling.

- Make sure you talk to your doctor or physical therapist first to find out if a sling is right for you.

Method 2. Stretching your Arms and Hands

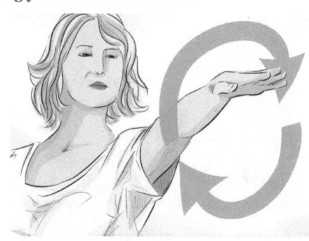

1. Rotate your arms. At least three times a day, move your arms through their full range of motion. Arm exercises will help your balance when you are walking as well as your ability to pick up and lift objects again.

- First, stretch out your affected arm until you can feel a slight burn. Hold it for 60 seconds (or as long as you are physically able) before relaxing.

- Make a wide circle with your arms. Go slowly, and try to reach out as far and high as you are able.

- Raise your arms above your head before lowering them. Repeat this motion at least five times. If you cannot raise your arm high, ask your physical therapist or caretaker to move it for you.

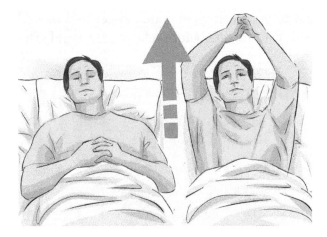

2. Improve shoulder motion. Lie on your back with your hands clasped beneath your breast. Gradually raise your arms until your clasped hands are above your shoulders. After a second, lower them back down again. Repeat five to ten times.

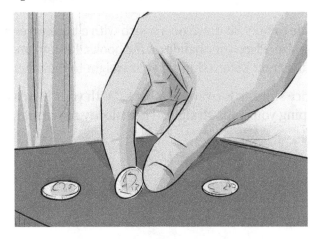

3. Pick up small objects. You can use pennies, marbles, pencils, or other small trinkets for this activity as long as you have a couple to work with. Pick up each small item with your affected hand, and place it in your unaffected hand. Hold them there until all of the small objects have been picked up. Next, take each object one by one out of the unaffected hand, and place them back in their original position.

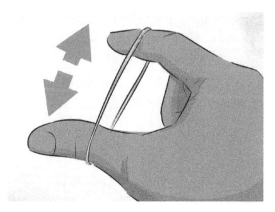

4. Exercise your hands with a rubber band. Loop a rubber band around one of your fingers and your thumb. You may want to start with your index finger and move back towards your pinky. Stretch the rubber band with your fingers before relaxing the band. This will help you regain fine motor control.

Method 3. Improving your Balance

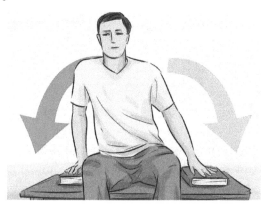

1. Shift your weight from side to side. Sit down on a bench with a book on either side of you. The books should be roughly the same size. Place your hands on the books. Lean to one side, shifting your weight to that side. Gently return to center before shifting your weight to the other side. Do this ten times.

- You can also practice shifting forward and back. With your hands on the books, gently lean forward while keeping your hips straight. Then slowly move into a small back lean.

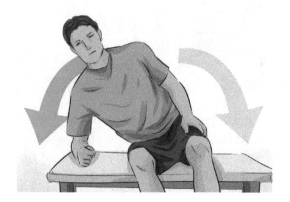

2. Lean on your elbows. Sit on a bench or firm bed. Lean on your arm so that your forearm is resting straight against the surface; you can place a pillow under your elbow if it hurts. With your hand, push down against the surface so that your arm straightens and your body rises. Slowly bend the elbow back down until you are in the original position.

- If you are having shoulder problems, do not try this exercise until you have strengthened your shoulder.

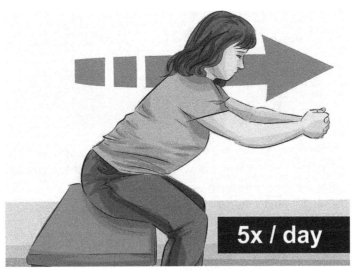

5x / day

3. Reach forward with your hands. While sitting on a firm chair, stretch your arms out in front of you and clasp your hands together. Lean forward slightly before straightening again. Try this five times every day until you have regained your balance.

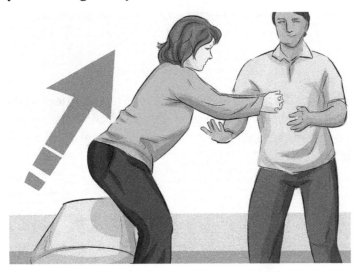

4. Practice moving from sitting to standing. When you are comfortable with leaning forward, you can try standing as you reach out. Keep your hands clasped, and slowly rise as high as you can from the chair. If you cannot stand completely yet, do not push yourself. Simply lower yourself back to the chair.

- Never try this unless you have someone there with you to catch you if you fall.

Method 4. Strengthening your Walking Muscles

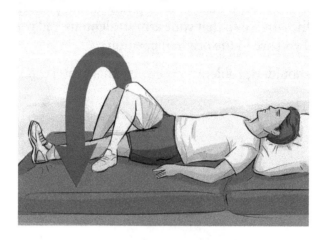

1. Stretch your hips. Lie on your back with your healthy leg stretched and your affected leg bent. Lift the affected leg, and move it over the other leg. Uncross your legs, returning the affected foot to its original position. Repeat five to ten times.

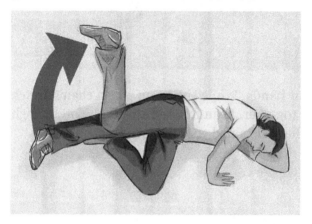

2. Practice walking while lying down. Lie down on the unaffected side of your body. The unaffected leg should be bent beneath your body to support your weight. Slowly bend your affected leg back so that your heel is reaching your backside before slowly straightening it back to its original position. Repeat five to ten times.

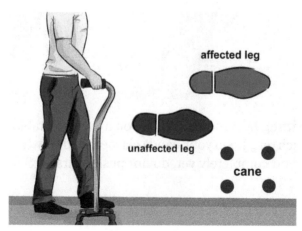

affected leg

unaffected leg

cane

3. Start walking with a cane. You may have to use a walking aid such as a cane or walker. Your physical therapist should train you how to use this before you leave the hospital. If not, invest in a cane with a rubber stopper on the end. Choose a grip that is comfortable. Hold the cane in the hand opposite your affected side. As you move your affected leg, move the cane forward as well. Keep the cane still when moving with your unaffected leg.

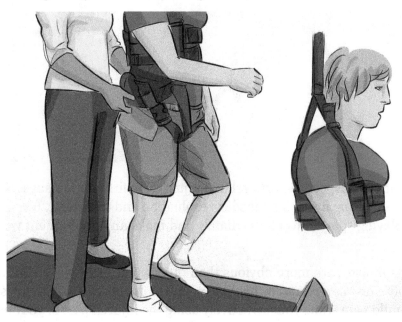

4. Walk on a treadmill. While being supervised by your physical therapist or caretaker, you can start walking on a treadmill to build strength and mobility back into your legs. Go at a very slow pace, and make sure you are holding onto the treadmill. Don't attempt to walk on the treadmill without supervision. Your physical therapist may recommend you use a weight support brace if you not yet able to keep your body upright for long.

- Your physical therapist may also recommend a stair climber if you are having difficulty lifting your legs or going up stairs. If you live in a place with stairs or steps, ask your therapist if this will be feasible for you.

How to use Physical Therapy to Recover from Sports Injuries

Rest and rehabilitation are essential to recovering from sports related injuries. If you've been injured playing sports, physical therapy can help maximize your chances of healing properly and getting back in the game. Start by getting your injuries evaluated and treated by a medical professional. Your healthcare provider may then refer you to a physical therapist. A physical therapist can prescribe exercises, stretches and a training regime that will help you to regain your strength quickly and fully. Take precautions to avoid injuring yourself again in the future.

Method 1. Having your Injuries Evaluated

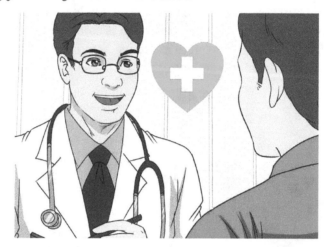

1. Go to the doctor if you suspect a sports-related injury. The first step to successfully recovering from a sports injury is getting immediate medical evaluation and treatment. If you hurt yourself or notice pain while playing sports, stop immediately and make an appointment with your primary care provider.

- Some sports injuries are more obvious than others. For example, a sprain or dislocation will probably cause severe and immediate pain. On the other hand, a stress fracture might only cause mild pain while you are actively using the injured part of your body.

- If you have experienced a serious injury, such as a head trauma, a broken bone, or a dislocation, go to the emergency department right away.

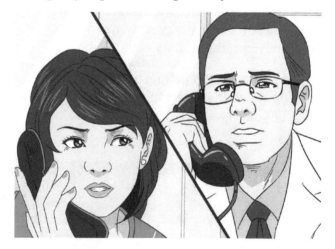

2. Find a therapist who specializes in sports injuries. If you play sports, you are likely to experience a range of common injuries associated with your specific sport. A therapist with experience treating these types of injuries will not only be able to diagnose and treat your injuries effectively, but can also help you master better technique and form so that future injuries will be less likely.

- For example, a physical therapist who is familiar with tennis elbow can prescribe exercises to strengthen the muscles in your arm and shoulder, and can also recommend equipment that will reduce stress on your elbow.

- Ask your primary care provider to recommend a physical therapist who specializes in sports injuries. If you have a coach or personal trainer, they may also be able to recommend someone.

- Check with your insurance company to make sure that the therapist and the facility you're interested in are in your network.

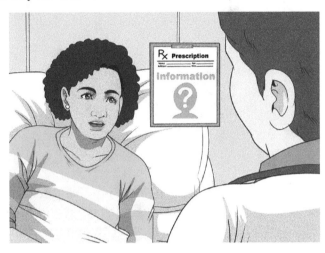

3. Provide your therapist with information about your injury. The type of physical therapy that is best for you will depend on the nature and severity of your injury. Provide your therapist with copies of any medical records relating to your injury, including medical images (such as X-rays).

- Tell your therapist when and how the injury occurred, and describe any symptoms you are experiencing (such as pain, swelling, or stiffness).

- Your therapist may also ask you for general health information, such as any medications you are currently taking and any history of health problems or previous injuries.

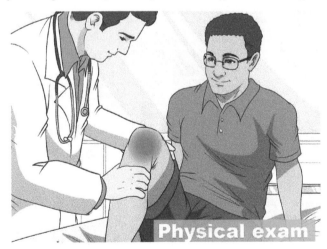

4. Allow your therapist to perform a physical exam. During your first meeting, your physical therapist will want to evaluate your injury and your overall physical state. They may also wish to observe you in motion performing activities related to your injury. Wear comfortable, loose-fitting clothing that allows easy access to the injured part of your body.

- For example, if you've sprained your knee, wear shorts. If you dislocated your shoulder, wear a tank top. Bring the shoes that you normally wear during sports activities.

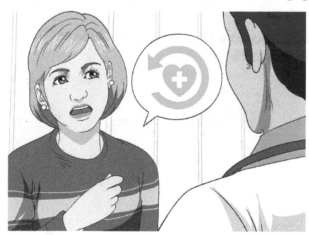

5. Discuss your recovery goals with your therapist. Your physical therapist can help you get a realistic sense of the ways in which physical therapy can help you, and how soon you can return to your regular activities. Talk to your therapist about what you hope to achieve, and ask if your goals are attainable.

- For example, you might say, "I'd like to get back to playing football within 6 months. Do you think that's doable."

- Your therapist will help you break your larger goals down into smaller, more specific goals. They will establish a timeframe for reaching these mini-goals, and help you design a process for reaching them (e.g., "Let's try these exercises, and work towards you being able to fully extend your elbow by the end of this week.").

Method 2. Establishing a Rehabilitation Routine

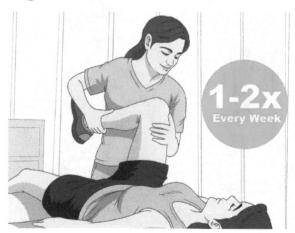

1. Go to therapy sessions as recommended by your therapist. Most physical therapy involves regular appointments with your therapist. Depending on the nature of your injuries, it may be necessary to meet with your therapist 1-2 times a week or as often as every day during the rehabilitation process.

- During these appointments, your therapist may help you do exercises and stretches, perform other types of therapy (such as massage), and assess your progress.

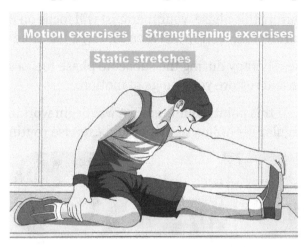

2. Do exercises at home following your therapist's suggestions. In addition to guiding you through stretches and exercises at their office, your physical therapist will prescribe therapeutic activities that you can do at home. Carefully follow all their instructions regarding technique, how often you should do the exercises, and for how long. Common types of at-home physical therapy exercises and techniques include:

- Range of motion exercises, which may involve gently flexing and extending a joint or moving an injured limb carefully in different directions.

- Strengthening exercises, which may involve using tools such as resistance bands or weights, or using your own body weight to create resistance.

- Static stretches, which can help improve circulation and relieve muscle tension and stiffness.

- Treatments to minimize pain and inflammation, such as using ice-packs or compression bandages.

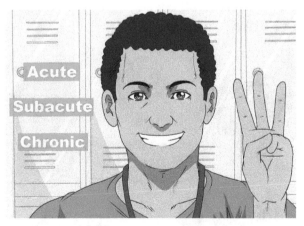

3. Adjust your rehabilitation routine as needed. Your rehabilitation program will need regular adjustment as you progress through the recovery process. Early sessions will probably focus mainly

on treating the injury, while later phases of the physical therapy process will be more geared toward building strength and restoring your range of motion. The 3 main phases of physical therapy are:

- The acute phase. During this phase, your therapist will focus on managing pain and inflammation, as well as protecting the injured area so that it has time to heal.

- The subacute phase. Therapy during the subacute phase focuses on helping you gradually strengthen the area and restore your range of motion.

- The chronic phase. At this point, your therapist will begin working on getting you prepared to return to your regular pre-injury activities and exercise routines.

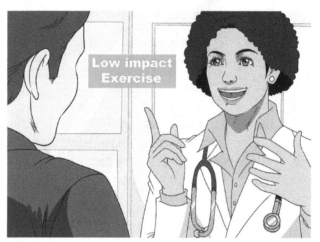

4. Ask your therapist about the best way to stay fit during recovery. During the early stages of recovery, it is important not to do anything that might slow your healing or make the injury worse. You will need to rest the injured part of your body and avoid returning to your regular activities too quickly. Your therapist can recommend low-impact exercises that will help you stay in shape without putting stress on your injury.

- For example, if you're a runner with a stress fracture in your foot, your physical therapist may recommend water jogging. This is a good form of low-impact cardiovascular exercise.

Method 3. Preventing Future Injuries

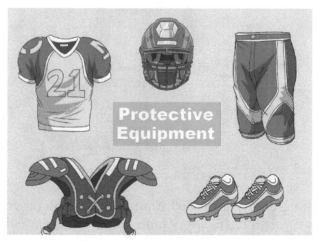

1. Wear proper protective equipment. Good safety equipment is crucial to preventing injury in many types of sports. Use all the recommended equipment for your sport, and check your equipment regularly to make sure it is not worn out or damaged.

- If you play a contact sport like hockey or football, you will need equipment such as shin pads, a helmet, and a face guard.

- High-quality, well-fitting shoes can also help prevent injury to your ankles, feet, and knees.

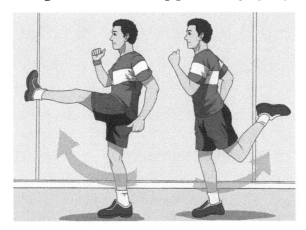

2. Do appropriate warm-ups. Warming up before sports or intense exercise is crucial for increasing joint and muscle flexibility and improving circulation. A proper warm-up should include dynamic stretches and light cardio activity, and should last at least 5 to 10 minutes.

- Dynamic stretches are stretches that you perform while moving, such as lunges and kicks. They are typically held for no longer than a few seconds.

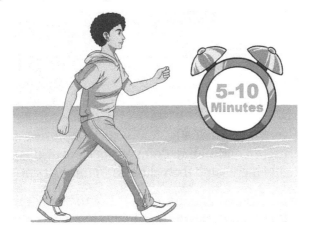

3. Cool down after playing sports. Cooling down after intense physical activity is important for minimizing stress on your heart and preventing stiffness and soreness. When you're done exercising or playing sports, cool down with 5 to 10 minutes of light exercise (such as a brisk walk) and do some static stretches to relax your muscles.

- Static stretches are stretches that you hold in a single position for 15 to 20 seconds. For example, you might perform a static hamstring stretch by sitting on the floor with 1 leg stretched out in front of you, then reaching out to touch your toes or your shin.

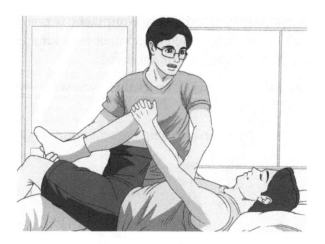

4. Work with a therapist, coach or trainer to improve your technique. You can prevent many common sports injuries by using proper technique. Your physical therapist, a coach, or a trainer can help you learn how to use your equipment properly and use your body correctly when you carry out specific movements or actions.

- For example, if you pitch in baseball, your physical therapist can show you how to use your shoulders, legs, and torso to reduce stress on your elbow when you pitch.

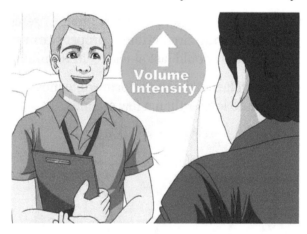

5. Ease into exercises and activities gradually. Many sports injuries, such as stress fractures or tendonitis, result from overuse. In addition to doing proper warm-ups, you can minimize the risk of overuse injuries by gradually increasing the volume and intensity of your exercise.

- Talk to your physical therapist about the best way to safely increase the amount and intensity of your exercise. A good rule of thumb is to increase your activity level by 10% each week until you reach your goal.

How to use Physical Therapy for Osteoporosis

Osteoporosis is a metabolic bone disease. This chronic condition results in weakened bone mass and fragility, often leading to bone fractures. Approximately 80 percent of osteoporosis patients are women over 50; however, this disease can affect men and women of any age. Many fractures occur in the spine, wrist and hips as a result of falling. Many people with osteoporosis become afraid to pursue physical activity. The risk of imbalance, falling and fracture can be lowered by using physical therapy as a treatment for osteoporosis. Physical therapy is also used to relieve pain and regain mobility after a fracture. Learn how to use physical therapy for osteoporosis.

Steps

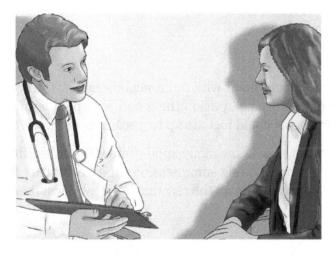

1. Visit your doctor to discuss physical therapy options. Physical therapy is used in conjunction with medication, braces or aides and regular tests. If you recently fractured a bone, your doctor may want you to wait 6 weeks, until you are in the sub-acute phase of your injury.

- If you have been diagnosed with osteoporosis, but you have not yet fractured a bone, you may need to approach your doctor about using physical therapy as a preventative measure. The physical therapist can teach you to move, exercise and even fall in a way that prevents serious and painful bone fractures.

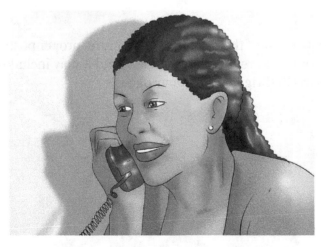

2. Choose a physical therapist that specializes in osteoporosis. The treatment regime for people who have lost bone mass is different from physical therapy used to treat other injuries. Ask your doctor for a list of specialized therapists.

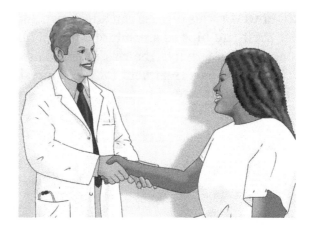

3. Schedule an evaluation appointment with a physical therapist. During this appointment, they will test your body mechanics, your physical fitness and your pain levels. The therapist will prescribe a treatment program that could include up to 3 sessions per week for 6 months.

• Talk to your therapist about how many appointments your health insurance will cover. In some cases, you can begin doing some sessions at a health care facility or gym. You may need to pay out of pocket to finish the recommended physical therapy program.

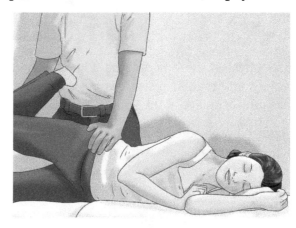

4. Learn proper posture. Because of the risk of spinal fracture, proper posture is essential to retaining mobility. Changing your posture is not always easy, and it may include exercises to strengthen muscles, braces or supports and vigilance on your part.

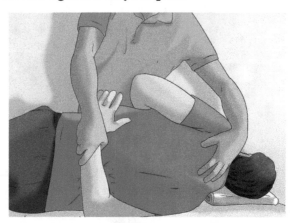

5. Change your body mechanics to fit your condition. For most people this means learning to lift properly, learning fall prevention, learning to avoid twisting your spine and asking for help with situations that could cause fractures (such as lifting or reaching). Your physical therapist will lead you through new movements that you can practice at home.

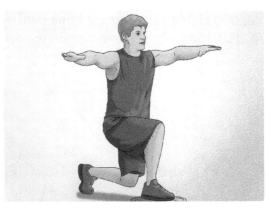

6. Do balance exercises. Exercises that teach you to walk steadily or balance on 1 foot (0.3 m) help you to avoid future falls. You may also be asked to do some light stretching, because this helps to increase range of motion in your joints and prevent falls.

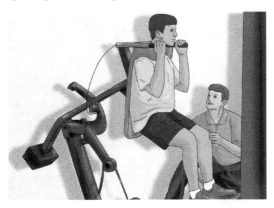

7. Begin weight-bearing exercises. This is any low-impact aerobic activity that requires you to move yourself around. Regular walking, dancing, elliptical and stair stepping machines all help to slow down mineral loss in your bones.

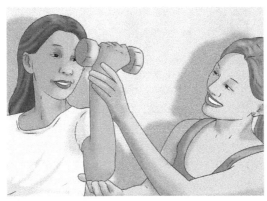

8. Start a strength-training routine. Under supervision by a physical therapist, do repetitive mo-

tions with small weights, resistance bands or weight machines in order to strengthen the muscles in your back and other parts of your body. Strength-training will increase the strength of the postural muscles and help you to avoid compression fractures, and stooping, along your spinal column.

- In healthy bodies, strength-training can increase bone density. In osteoporosis patients, exercises with weight or resistance help you to maintain your current bone mass and avoid future loss of bone density.

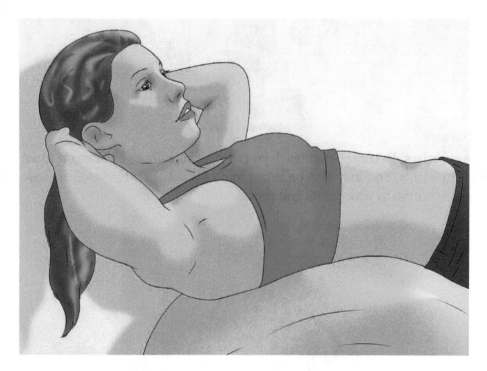

9. Begin your own preventative exercise routine at home, after 1 to 6 months of physical therapy. This should include weight-bearing, strength-training and balance exercise almost every day. Regular, careful physical activity should be taken as seriously as taking an osteoporosis medication.

How to use Physical Therapy to Relieve Arthritis Symptoms

Those with arthritis who use physical therapy, or PT, as part of their treatment regimen report lessened symptoms, less pain, better sleep, and greater mobility. Physical therapy usually consists of range of motion exercises, strengthening exercises, and low-impact aerobic exercises. You should begin physical therapy with a professional physical therapist, and continue your treatment at home. It is important to personalize your PT plan to target your symptoms and avoid an increase in pain. With a little dedication and persistence, you can use physical therapy to help decrease the symptoms of your arthritis.

Method 1. Using Range of Motion Exercises

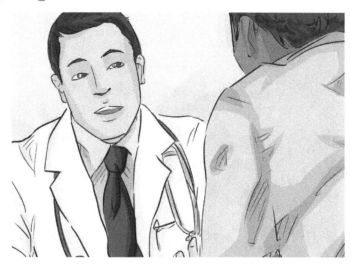

1. Learn about the benefits of range of motion exercises. These exercises are prescribed by physical therapists to help your joints go through their full range of motion. They also help relieve stiffness.

- Range of motion exercises typically involve rotating a certain joint all the way around several times to strengthen the joint.

2. Do arm circles. Try holding 1 arm out to the side and begin rotating it forward in a circular motion. Start by doing large circles, and then transition to smaller circles. This will help improve mobility in your shoulder joints.

- You can also try rotating other joints – like your ankles and wrists.

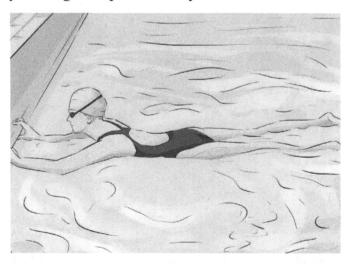

3. Try water exercises. Consider beginning range of motion exercises in water, as the more weightless environment puts less initial strain on your body. You can practice reaching your arms forward in the water, rotating your wrist and finger joints, or even bending your elbows.

- Try arm circles while you are in the water. This will make these exercises even gentler on your body.

- You could also take a water aerobics class. Your physical therapist may be able to recommend one for you.

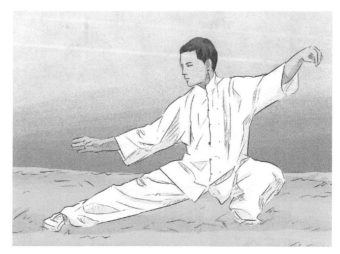

4. Learn tai-chi. You can also do tai-chi to improve range of motion and balance. The gentle, fluid motions are perfect exercises for joints with arthritis. And the low-impact nature of tai-chi is great for people of all ages.

- Try joining a tai-chi class at a local gym or physical therapy center. You can also try following along with a tai-chi video at home, if you feel comfortable learning the routines without the help of an instructor.

Method 2. Doing Strengthening Exercises

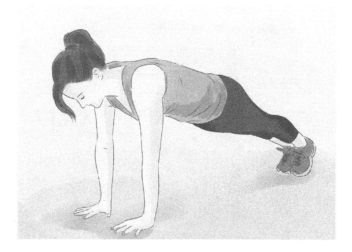

1. Benefit from strengthening exercises. Improving muscle strength actually increases bone density, an important element with arthritis and osteoporosis. Your physical therapist will teach you isometric exercises, which rely on keeping a muscle or group of muscles in a static, flexed position. This means that the exercises are done in a single position without movement.

- Isotonic exercise works by using your body weight or small weights to help you build muscle mass.

- When done properly these exercises add stability to your joints and decrease pain.

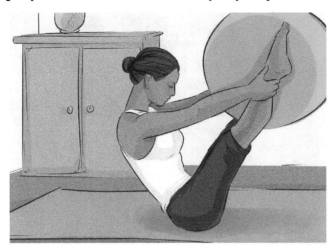

2. Use an exercise ball. Ask your physical therapist to teach you how to use an exercise ball correctly to prevent injuries. Using an exercise ball can help strengthen your core, increase balance, and decrease pain. Just sitting on an exercise ball can improve core strength. You can also lie on the exercise ball on your stomach while alternating between lifting each leg.

- You can use different sized balls for different exercises.

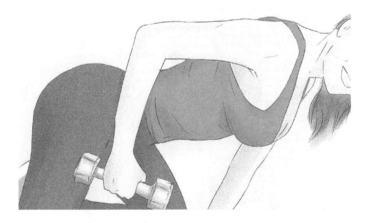

3. Strengthen your muscles and joints by using weights. Try using free weights or a weight machine to improve your mobility and ease joint pain. Focus on lighter weights with more repetitions rather than adding on extra weight. This will help you avoid a flare up of your arthritis symptoms.

- If your arthritis is particularly bad, use machines without any added weight, such as doing exercises with a barbell.

- Speak to your physical therapist about the right amount of weight to use and the best number of repetitions for your specific case. Generally, you could to 2-3 sets of 15 reps.

- Be careful not to overdo it when you are using the weights. You don't want to push your body too hard.

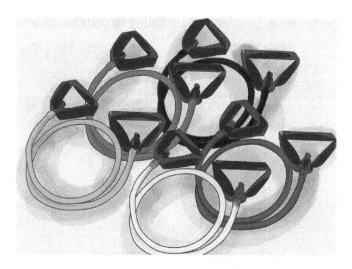

4. Use resistance bands. Ask your physical therapist to teach you how to use a resistance band before trying these exercises. Resistance bands are pieces of rubber that you can use while exercising that help strengthen your muscles and joints. They work by adding additional resistance to the movements you are already doing.

- Try looping the resistance band around your foot and pulling it toward you with both arms.

- Try positioning the resistance band around your elbow and flexing your arm up while holding the resistance band in the hand of the same arm.

Method 3. Trying Appropriate Aerobic Exercises

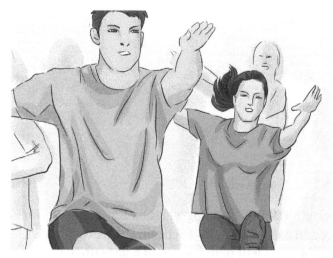

1. Start doing low or medium intensity aerobic exercise. Most arthritis sufferers are recommended to do pool therapy. You can attend water aerobics classes, do water walking, or learn a water therapy routine with your physical therapist.

- This is a crucial element of physical therapy if you need to lose weight. It will increase endurance and improve daily function.

- Some centers or gyms have classes specifically for people suffering from arthritis.

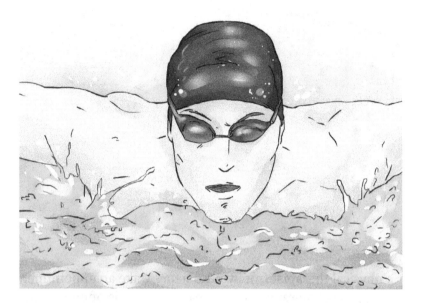

2. Start swimming. In addition to other water aerobic routines, you can try some low-impact swimming. Take a few easy laps around the pool if you're able to. This can really help minimize your symptoms of arthritis.

- Try some slow breast strokes, or even just floating on your back for a few minutes at a time.

- You can also sit in a Jacuzzi or hot tub with jets, which may help mobilize your joints.

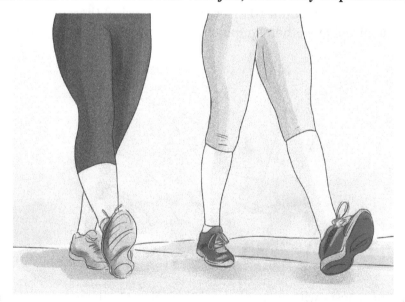

3. Try walking. Walking is a great way to remain active in your daily life. Take a nice stroll around your neighborhood, or find a track nearby that you can walk.

- Make sure you don't push yourself too hard or walk for longer than your body can handle.

- You could also try bicycling as an alternative to walking. Both outdoor biking and riding an indoor stationary bike can help reduce your arthritis symptoms.

Method 4. Starting a Physical Therapy Program

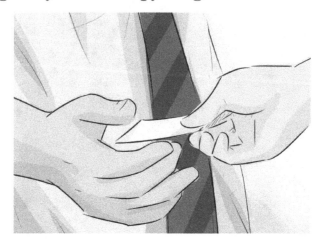

1. Get a referral for a physical therapist from your doctor. Make an appointment with your doctor to discuss exercise and physical therapy. PT is a treatment that is often prescribed by your doctor and covered by insurance. Discuss your current pain and mobility problems and create a general exercise plan.

- You may find that a therapist is used to treating people with osteoarthritis, rheumatoid arthritis, or elderly or younger patients. They may also specialize in a specific anatomical area, such as the knees or back.

- Take the facilities into account when choosing a physical therapist. Look for a center that has a water pool and any other equipment you may need.

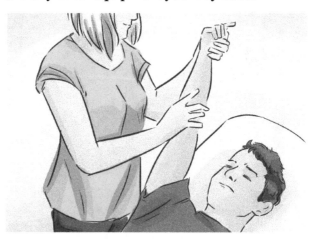

2. Undergo preliminary tests with your physical therapist. Go through an evaluation with your physical therapist before you get started with exercises or other therapies. The physical therapist will test muscle strength, mobility, pain, and body mechanics. Ask your physical therapist to write down a plan based on the results.

- Ask your physical therapist if weight loss would possibly ease your symptoms. If you are overweight and have arthritis in your ankles, knees, back and shoulders, then weight loss should be one of your primary physical therapy goals.

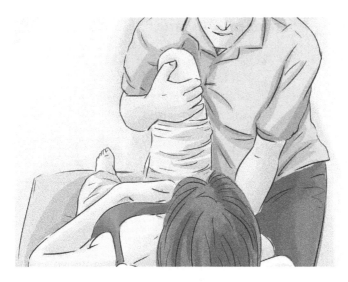

3. Continue with your physical therapy schedule. Plan to visit the physical therapist as often as they recommend. In many cases, your insurance may only cover appointments twice per week for a few months. Ask your doctor to write you a letter overriding these limits so your insurance will cover more appointments. Regular meetings can help to relieve more symptoms of arthritis and mobility issues than occasional sessions.

- In many cases, patients need to increase their muscle mass, which can only be done with regular exercise.

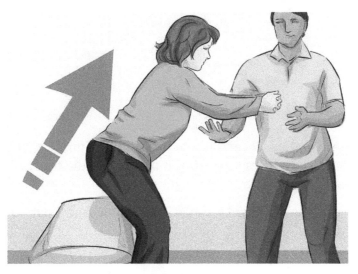

4. Learn proper body mechanics. Before beginning to exercise, the therapist will make sure that you can get out of bed, get up from a chair, and walk without putting undue pressure on your joints. The therapist will teach you how to change your body mechanics, if necessary.

- Use aides as prescribed by your physical therapist. If you are unable to perform regular day-to-day motions without increasing the stress on your joints, you may be prescribed a cane, walker, sock gripper, shower stool, or other device. Use them as directed, and you may notice a gradual decrease in your pain.

Method 5. Continuing Treatment at Home

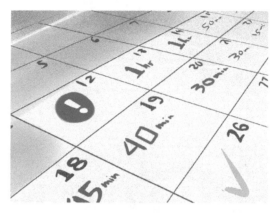

1. Develop a weekly exercise plan. Muscles support the joints, and an unused muscle can quickly lose its function. Create a weekly exercise routine that you can do from home, or at least unassisted.

- Stick to your exercise routine. The more consistent you are, the more it will help your arthritis symptoms.

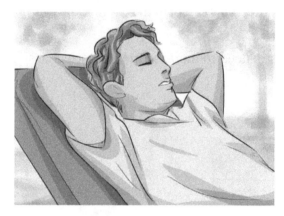

2. Use rest to treat active symptoms. Learn how to treat arthritis properly at home. Your doctor has likely prescribed non-steroidal anti-inflammatories or other medicine. However, you may want to use rest as your first line of defense against arthritis symptoms.

- Get to know your signs of fatigue. Lay flat on a bed or take a nap to reduce stress on your back or other joints.

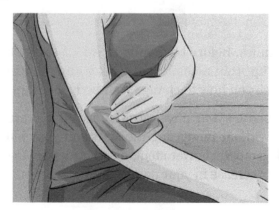

3. Apply ice and heat. Ice should be used to treat inflammation and numb pain, as tolerated. It is especially effective if you have a new, acute injury. Moist heat should be used to treat muscle spasms. Take a hot shower or use a microwavable heat pack for 20 minutes to treat symptoms.

- Remember that overuse of heat can increase inflammation.

- Your physical therapist may use an ultrasound machine for heat therapy while you are in the office.

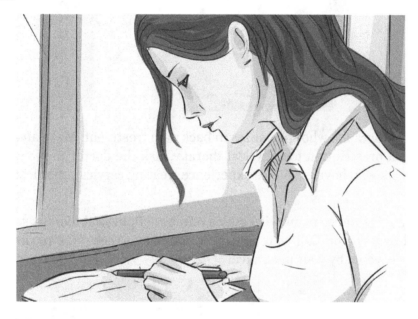

4. Build a physical therapy routine that you can do at home. Physical therapy will not end once you stop going to sessions; it is intended to change your lifestyle so that you can become more active. Create a weekly plan that is feasible within your current schedule.

- You may also need some adaptations in your home like a shower stool or shower bars. These can help you minimize the impact of your arthritis symptoms in your daily life.

- Ask your physical therapist to come to your home to assess your needs and suggest equipment that may be helpful.

How to use Physical Therapy to Relieve Back Pain

Researchers estimate that between 90 and 95 percent of adults suffer from acute back pain at some point in their lives. The treatments for back pain include rest, injections, ice, pain medication and even surgery. For the majority of injuries, doctors have moved away from prescribing bed rest and moved towards a rehabilitative exercise routine. One of the ways to safely and successfully create an exercise routine is to schedule regular sessions with a physical therapist. Therapists work to retrain your posture, strengthen your core and stretch tight muscles. Learn how to use physical therapy to relieve back pain.

Steps

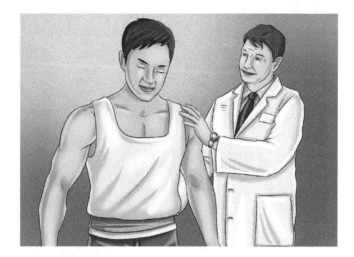

1. Choose a physical therapist who specializes in back pain treatment. Make an appointment with your doctor to get a prescription for physical therapy. Ask the doctor to recommend a handful of physical therapists who have extensive experience treating cervical, thoracic or lumbar spinal pain.

- Many private insurance plans will cover a number of physical therapy sessions, if they are prescribed by a doctor. Call your insurance company to see if the recommended physical therapist is covered by your insurance.

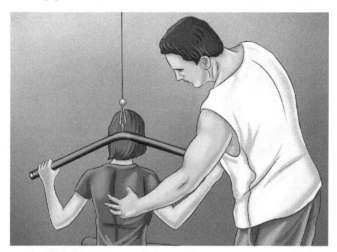

2. Wait until you are at the sub-acute stage of injury before you start physical therapy. There are 3 stages of injury: acute, sub-acute and chronic stages. The sub-acute phase usually begins 2 to 4 weeks after injury.

- During the acute stage you should avoid bending, lifting, stooping and prolonged sitting. Most doctors recommend a treatment of non-steroidal anti-inflammatory pills and ice for the first few days after a back injury. After the first few days, try to avoid bed rest and return to a more normal activity level. Walking and gentle stretching can help to increase circulation and improve healing.

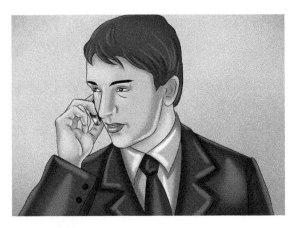

3. Schedule an evaluation with your physical therapist. The first session will be dedicated to strength, balance and pain level tests. Your therapist should design a program based on your strengths and weaknesses.

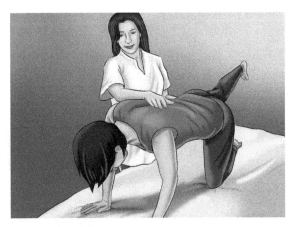

4. Learn and practice proper posture. Physical therapists are starting to use global postural re-education (GPR) to assist patients in developing proper posture. PT techniques will include assisted stretching, range of motion exercises and muscle strengthening exercises.

- Changing your posture requires diligence for weeks and months. Your physical therapist may prescribe daily stretches and exercise to retrain muscles.

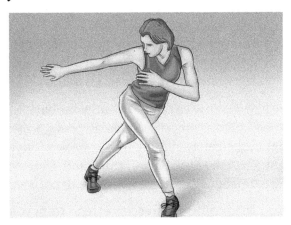

5. Begin low-impact aerobic exercise. This includes walking, swimming or using an elliptical. These

activities cause very little stress on your back, while toning and stretching muscles and increasing circulation.

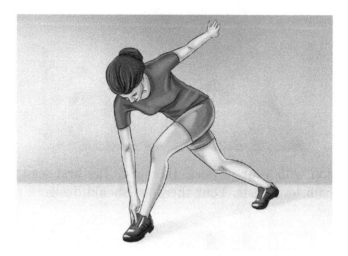

6. Start your aerobic exercise routine gradually. Your physical therapist may give you some methods to try, such as doing a 10-minute elliptical warm up before stretching or exercising. Increase the exercise in small increments to avoid further injury and pain. As your muscles get stronger, you should be able to be more active without increasing your pain.

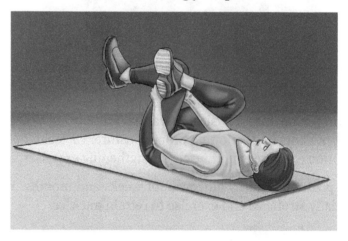

7. Begin a regular stretching routine. People often complain of "sciatica" or pain caused by the sciatic nerve through the hips, buttocks and legs. This, and other back problems, can be lessened dramatically by doing back and leg stretching once or twice daily.

- Do hamstring stretches once or twice daily. Lay on your back with your knees up. Lift and gently pull 1 knee into your chest for 10 seconds. Repeat 3 times on each side. Follow this stretch with the straight leg stretch. While on your back with your knees bent, lift 1 leg so that it is nearly straight. Grab the back of your thigh and bring it toward you for 10 seconds. Try to keep your leg as straight as possible. Repeat with both legs 3 times.

- Do piriformis stretches. The piriformis muscles extend from your lower back through your buttocks and hips. While on your back with your knees bent, raise your right leg and rotate it to the left. Place your right leg on your left thigh just above your right ankle. Grasp your left thigh and bring it toward you. Hold for 30 seconds. Repeat twice on each side.

- Do the child's pose. This yoga stretch works on the back, leg and buttock muscles. Lay on your stomach. Place your hands underneath your shoulders and fold your body back so your knees touch the front of your torso. Reach your hands out in front of your head as far as you can. Hold this stretch for 1 to 5 minutes.

- Do other stretches as recommended by your physical therapist. The evaluation should show which muscles are the tightest.

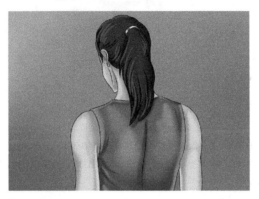

8. Begin a strengthening exercise routine 3 to 4 times per week. These exercises should target your underlying core and postural muscles. When these muscles are strong, they support the spine and lower pain.

- Lay on your back with your knees bent. Press your back into the floor. Hold for 10 seconds. Release and rest for 3 seconds. Repeat 10 to 20 times. Pelvic tilts help to strengthen back and stomach muscles.

- Do swimming. Lay on your stomach with your legs and arms outstretched. Raise 1 arm, hold for 3 seconds and lower it slowly. Repeat on the opposite side. Repeat 10 times with your arms and 10 times with your legs. Once your muscles get used to arms and legs separately, do the exercise with opposite legs and arms.

- Do shoulder squeezes. While standing or sitting, lower your shoulders and squeeze your shoulder blades together as much as possible. Hold for 3 seconds and slowly release. Repeat 10 times. Do this whenever your shoulders are feeling stiff or you have spare time.

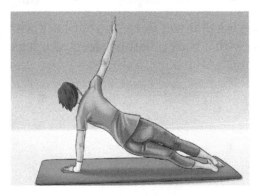

9. Create an exercise space at home so that you can do your exercises. Buy a yoga mat, small

weights and any other low-cost equipment you use at physical therapy. You can reduce your sessions with a physical therapist if you are committed to doing the physical therapy routine at home.

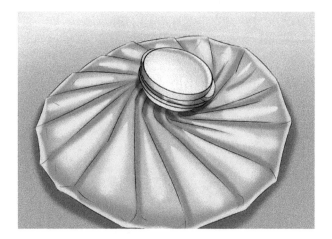

10. Use pain treatment modalities. These are usually done at the end of a physical therapy session. Your physical therapist may suggest ice to reduce swelling, moist heat for muscle spasms or ultrasound for increasing circulation.

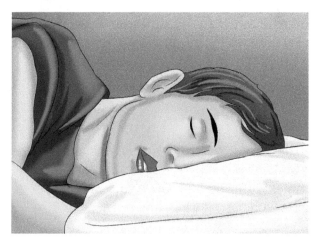

11. Get plenty of rest. Success in physical therapy requires that you avoid sitting or standing too much. Focus on getting plenty of sleep and keeping your back straight at night.

- Physical therapists suggest that you sleep on your back with your knees propped up with pillows or on your side with a body pillow between your legs.

Massage Therapy: A Significant Aspect of Physical Therapy

Massage is the manual manipulation of the body using fingers, hands, knees, elbows, feet or any device. It is done for the treatment of stress or pain and for general health and well-being. The topics elaborated in this chapter will help in gaining a better perspective about the significant aspects of physical therapy and the ways to start a massage therapy business and become a massage therapist. It also explores the techniques of delivering effective hot stone massage, full body massage, leg massage, etc.

Massage therapy is the scientific manipulation of the soft tissues of the body, consisting primarily of manual (hands-on) techniques such as applying fixed or movable pressure, holding, and moving muscles and body tissues.

Purpose

Generally, massage is delivered to improve the flow of blood and lymph (fluid in lymph glands, part of immune system), to reduce muscular tension or flaccidity, to affect the nervous system through stimulation or sedation, and to enhance tissue healing. Therapeutic massage may be recommended for children and adults to deliver benefits such as the following:

- Reducing muscle tension and stiffness
- Relieving muscle spasms
- Increasing joint and limb flexibility and range of motion
- Increasing ease and efficiency of movement
- Relieving points of tension and overall stress; inducing relaxation
- Promoting deeper and easier breathing
- Improving blood circulation and movement of lymph
- Relieving tension-related headaches and eyestrain
- Promoting faster healing of soft tissue injuries, such as pulled muscles and sprained ligaments
- Reducing pain and swelling related to injuries
- Reducing the formation of scar tissue following soft tissue injuries
- Enhancing health and nourishment of skin
- Improving posture by changing tension patterns that affect posture

- Reducing emotional or physical stress and reducing anxiety

- Promoting feelings of well-being

- Increasing awareness of the mind-body connection and improving mental awareness and alertness generally.

Massage therapy may also be recommended for its documented clinical benefits such as improving pulmonary function in young asthma patients, reducing psychoemotional distress in individuals who suffer from chronic inflammatory bowel disease, helping with weight gain, improving motor development in premature infants, and enhancing immune system functioning.

Description

Massage therapy is one of the oldest healthcare practices known. References to massage are found in ancient Chinese medical texts written more than 4,000 years ago. Massage has been advocated in Western healthcare practices since the time of Hippocrates, the "father of medicine."

Massage therapy is the scientific manipulation of the soft tissues of the body for the purpose of normalizing those tissues and consists of a group of manual techniques that include applying fixed or movable pressure, holding, and/or causing movement to parts of the body. While massage therapy is applied primarily with the hands, sometimes the forearms or elbows are used. These techniques affect the muscular, skeletal, circulatory, lymphatic, nervous, and other systems of the body. The basic philosophy of massage therapy embraces the concept of *vis Medicatrix naturae* , which means "aiding the ability of the body to heal itself."

Touch is the fundamental medium of massage therapy. While massage can be described in terms of the type of techniques performed, touch is not used solely in a mechanistic way in massage therapy. Because massage usually involves applying touch with some degree of pressure and movement, the massage therapist must use touch with sensitivity in order to determine the optimal amount of pressure to use for each person. For example, using too much pressure may cause the body to tense up, while using too little may not have enough effect. Touch used with sensitivity also allows the massage therapist to receive useful information via his or her hands about the individual's body, such as locating areas of muscle tension and other soft tissue problems. Because touch is also a form of communication, sensitive touch can convey a sense of caring to the person receiving massage, enhancing the individual's sense of self and well being.

In practice, many massage therapists use more than one technique or method in their work and sometimes combine several. Effective massage therapists ascertain each person's needs and then use the techniques that will best meet those needs.

Swedish massage is the most commonly used form of massage. It uses a system of long gliding strokes, kneading, and friction techniques on the more superficial layers of muscles, generally in the direction of blood flow toward the heart, and sometimes combined with active and passive movements of the joints. It is used to promote general relaxation, improve circulation and range of motion, and relieve muscle tension.

Deep tissue massage is used to release chronic patterns of muscular tension using slow strokes, direct pressure, or friction directed across the grain of the muscles. It is applied with greater pressure and to deeper layers of muscle than Swedish, which is why it is called deep tissue and is effective for chronic muscular tension.

Sports massage uses techniques that are similar to Swedish and deep tissue but are specially adapted to deal with the effects of athletic performance on the body and the needs of athletes regarding training, performing, and recovery from injury.

Neuromuscular massage is a form of deep massage that is applied to individual muscles. It is used primarily to release trigger points (intense knots of muscle tension that refer pain to other parts of the body) and also to increase blood flow. It is often used to reduce pain. Trigger point massage and myotherapy are similar forms.

Acupressure applies finger or thumb pressure to specific points located on the energy pathways or "meridians" in order to release blocked energy along these meridians that may be causing physical discomfort. The rebalance of energy flow releases tension and restores function of organs and muscles in the body. Shiatsu is a Japanese form of acupressure that applies these principles.

Massage therapy sessions can be at home or in a professional office. Most sessions are one hour. Frequency of massage sessions can vary widely as needed based on the condition being treated. The cost of massage therapy varies according to geographic location, experience of the massage therapist, and length of the massage. In the United States, as of 2004, the average range is from $35 to $60 for a one-hour session.

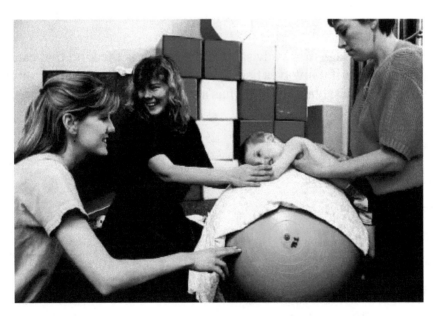

The first appointment generally begins with information gathering, such as the reason for getting massage therapy, physical condition and medical history, and other areas. The client is asked to remove clothing to one's level of comfort. Undressing takes place in private, and a sheet or towel is provided for draping. The massage therapist will undrape only the part of the body being massaged. The individual's modesty is respected at all times. The massage therapist may use an oil or cream, which is quickly absorbed into the skin.

Insurance coverage for massage therapy varies widely. There tends to be greater coverage in states that license massage therapy. In most cases, a physician's prescription for massage therapy is needed. Once massage therapy is prescribed, authorization from the insurer may be needed if coverage is not clearly spelled out in one's policy or plan.

Massage therapy may be recommended for children to help relieve conditions such as allergies , anxietyand stress, arthritis, asthma and bronchitis , joint or limb injuries, post-surgical muscle rehabilitation, chronic and temporary pain, circulatory problems, depression, digestive disorders, tension headaches, sleep problems or insomnia, myofascial pain, sports injuries , and eating problems associated with temporomandibular joint dysfunction.

Precautions

Massage is comparatively safe; however, it should not be used if the child has one of the following conditions.

- Advanced heart disease
- Hypertension (high blood pressure)
- Phlebitis
- Thrombosis
- Embolism
- Kidney failure

If the child has cancer , massage is not advisable if the cancer is the kind that can spread to other organs (metastatic cancer) or if it involves tissue damage due to chemotherapy or other treatment. Massage may also not be advisable if the child has any of the following conditions.

- A cold
- An infectious disease
- a contagious skin conditions
- An acute inflammation
- An infected injuries
- An unhealed fractures
- Dislocations
- Is postoperative with a condition in which pain and muscular splinting are increased
- Has frostbite
- Has large hernias
- Has torn ligaments
- Has any condition prone to hemorrhage

- Has a psychosis
- Has any other psychological state that may impair communication or perception

Massage should not be used locally on affected areas (i.e., avoid using massage on the specific areas of the body that are affected by the condition) for the following conditions: eczema, goiter (thyroid dysfunction), and open skin lesions. Massage may be used on the areas of the body that are not affected by these conditions. The decision to use massage must be based on whether it may cause harm. A physician's recommendation is appropriate before a child with any health condition receives massage therapy.

Preparation

Going for a massage requires little in the way of preparation. Generally, one should be clean and should not eat just before a massage. Massage therapists generally work by appointment and usually provide information about how to prepare for an appointment. To receive the most benefit from a massage, parents should give the therapist accurate health information about the child and report discomfort of any kind (whether it is from the massage itself or due to the room temperature or any other distractions). The child can be encouraged to be as receptive to the process as possible.

Aftercare

There are no special recommendations for after a massage. A period of quiet activity or rest following the massage helps maintain full benefits from the procedure.

Risks

Massage therapy does not have notable side effects. Rather than feeling too relaxed or too mentally unfocused after a massage, a child may be both more relaxed and more alert.

Parental Concerns

Parents who may not have experienced therapeutic massage themselves or who have doubts about its effectiveness may be interested in the results of research studies, particularly those conducted on groups of children. Well designed studies have documented the benefits of massage therapy for the treatment of acute and chronic pain, acute and chronic inflammation, chronic lymphedema, nausea , muscle spasm, various soft tissue dysfunctions, anxiety, depression, insomnia, and psychoemotional stress, which may aggravate mental illness.

How to Become a Massage Therapist

Massage therapy helps millions of people cope with physical ailments, sore muscles, and emotional distress. If you have a gift for giving a wonderful massage, becoming a professional massage therapist could be a great career opportunity and a way to truly help other people with your skill.

Part 1. Gaining Massage Experience

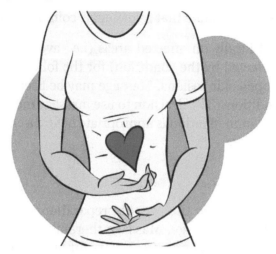

1. Figure out if your heart's in the right place. You might be good with your hands, but are you also patient and empathetic? Massage therapists need to be concerned about other people's holistic wellbeing. Receiving a massage is a very intimate experience. A good massage therapist respects that the art of massage is both physical and emotional.

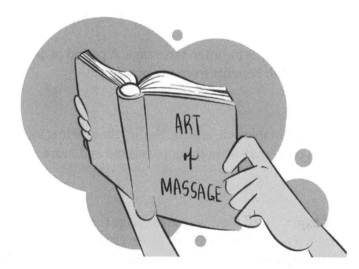

2. Learn about the art of massage. A great way to learn more about the massage arts is to talk with a massage therapist, and get a massage yourself. Ask plenty of questions about what the profession entails, and start thinking about what type of massage therapist you want to be.

- Do some research. Look online for information about different types of massage, or check out massage books at your local library. You can learn a lot about massage therapy just by reading about it.

- Practice on friends. Start getting a feel for what your "bedside manner" should be like, and how a typical session should go.

3. Consider specializing. There are many specialties in massage therapy and most massage therapists concentrate on one or more of these, especially when starting out. Different types of mas-

sage are used to different ends; some are geared toward healing muscles, some toward easing stress, and others toward helping with specific physical ailments. While you can, and probably will, learn more than one massage style, it's a good idea to think about what you're most interested in so that you can be sure to get appropriate training. Here are a few different types of massage to look into:

- Sports massage. This form of massage is designed to help athletes recover from injuries and everyday play, allowing them to perform at their physical best at the next game.

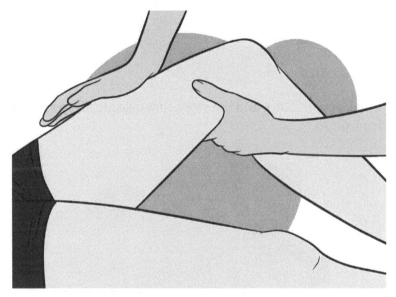

- Clinical massage. This focuses on using massage to heal physical ailments. A thorough understanding of anatomy is required.

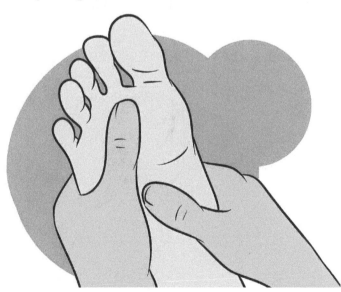

- Swedish massage. This is the most common type of massage, and is used for both healing and relaxation purposes. Deep tissue massage is a similar form of massage, but more pressure is exerted on the muscles.

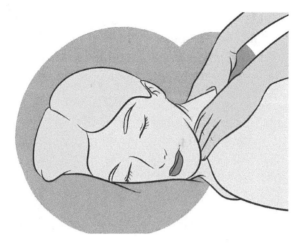

- Reflexology, reiki, acupressure, and hot stone massage are all special types of massage that serve specific purposes.

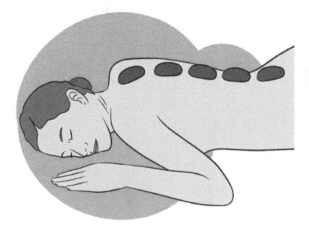

Part 2. Getting Licensed and Certified

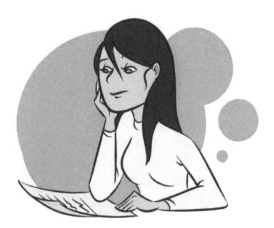

1. Research your jurisdiction's licensing requirements. Before you start training, it's a good idea to make sure that you understand how to satisfy your jurisdiction's licensing requirements so you'll know what kind of training will qualify you to be licensed.

- In the U.S. most states have some form of licensing, so check with your state's licensing board to get more information. Keep in mind that even if your state does not have licensing requirements, your city or county may.

- Some jurisdictions require licensing for some types of massage but not for others.

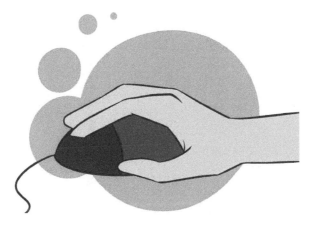

2. Find a suitable training program. There are plenty of massage schools out there. You may have seen their ads or even received advertising materials for some of them. Keep in mind that these schools are businesses that are trying to make money, so be sure to check out all their claims carefully. Look for a program that leads to certification and which satisfies your jurisdiction's licensing requirements, which may include accreditation.

- Most massage schools teach basic Swedish massage and allow you to choose other specialties in addition to that. Look for a school that caters to any specialties you are most interested in.

- You can research schools online, or you can ask massage therapists what schools they went to and what they thought of their experiences.

- You'll also want to consider your budget. Massage schools can be quite expensive, with tuition ranging from a few thousand dollars to tens of thousands. Most schools offer some kind of financial assistance, including federal student loans.

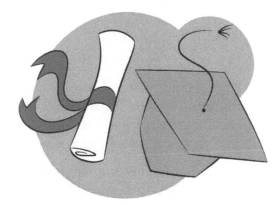

3. Complete your training program: In the U.S., many states require at least 500-600 hours of

training, so you can expect to spend at least that much time in the classroom and practicing. You can find a range of course lengths. How long it takes you to complete the program will depend on how many classes you take at one time; how quickly you complete your "practice" massages, and what your specialty is. Depending on the program you take, you will graduate either with certification in a certain specialty or with a degree.

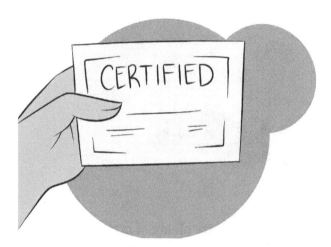

4. Consider Getting certified: Not all jurisdictions require certification, but becoming board certified can open a lot of doors for you. In the U.S. the National Certification Board of Massage Therapy administers an exam-based certification program. National Certification is not really needed unless it is required by your state for licensing.

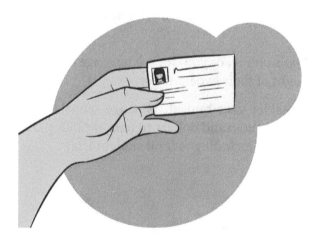

5. Get licensed: As mentioned before, you may need to become licensed in your jurisdiction. Your school should be able to assist you in understanding the licensing requirements and obtaining your license. National Certification is required by some states in the U.S., while others do not require it, and others require their own professional licensing exam.

- Many states are now accepting another exam offered by the Federation of Massage State Boards, which could lead to National Certification becoming obsolete.

- If you plan to start your own business, you will also most likely need to also get a business license from your state or municipality before you can practice.

- business license from your state or municipality before you can practice.

Part 3. Practicing as a Massage Therapist

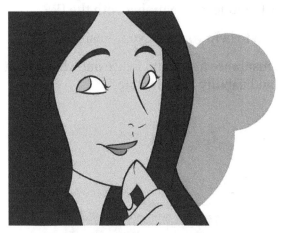

1. Decide whether to start your own business or look for a job. In the past, just about all massage therapists worked for themselves. Now there are a growing number of salaried jobs in massage therapy at massage parlors, spas, hotels, and other establishments, so you have a lot of options. Most jobs are low paying and start at $15 an hour, but you can find some jobs that pay much more than that.

- While you can usually make more money starting your own business, it can be difficult to get clients at first, and business expenses can pile up. If you want to start your own business, you'll need to lease a space in a central location to pick up plenty of clients.

- Another option is to contract with a health care provider or group of massage therapists to share a space. You'd still be in charge of your own services and business, but you'd have more security operating out of an established.

- Your massage school should be able to provide some counseling to help you make your choice.

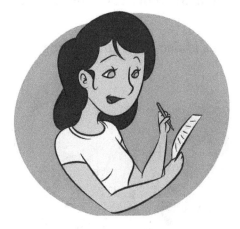

2. Take care of business items. Setting up a massage business is similar to setting up other types of small businesses. In order to legally operate as a business, there are certain requirements you must follow:

- Pick a business name and get it registered.

- File incorporation documents with the state.

- Apply for an Employer Identification Number with the IRS.

- Get a small business loan to help you start your business.

- Get insurance. Call an insurance agent and figure out what insurance you'll need to protect you from malpractice and liability in your state.

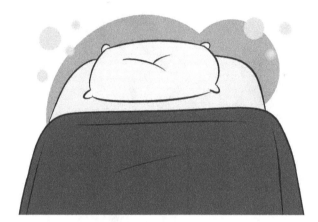

3. Set up your massage space. If you're running your own business, you'll be in charge of setting up the space. It's important for it to be extremely clean as well as welcoming and warm, so your clients feel comfortable spending time there. Here's what you'll need to do:

- Purchase equipment. You'll need a massage table, chair, pillows, sheets, lotions, oils, and any equipment you may need for the specialized type of massage services you're offering.

- Create a relaxing atmosphere. Have candles, light dimmers, or soft natural lighting in your space. Paint the walls a soothing earth tone, and hang calming art on the walls.

- You may want to offer a changing room and a place for clients to store their belongings during the session.

- Make sure the bathroom area is also clean and calming.

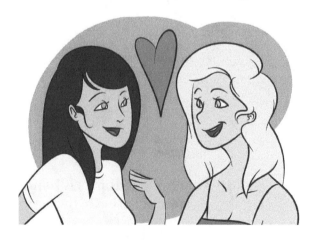

4. Market your services: The field of massage arts is growing, so it's important to find ways to set yourself apart from other massage therapists. What is it about you or your business that makes you unique and appealing? Spread the word about your business in the following ways:

- Use social media. Create a Facebook page and a Twitter account to announce deals and other news.

- Take out a local advertisement. Put yourself on the map by advertising in a local weekly newspaper.

- Have a grand opening event. Offer a tour of the facilities and a discount to people who come to the party. Don't forget to serve refreshments!

- Provide excellent service. The best way to get more clients is to do a wonderful job with the first few, so people will start recommending you to their friends.

How to Choose a Massage Course

Having a hard time finding the perfect massage course for you? Doing your own due diligence work can save you a lot of time and money. Here is what you need to look for.

Steps

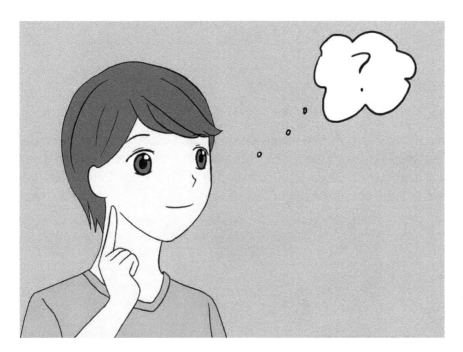

1. Why do you want to learn massage? There are many different motives for attending a massage course including a) personal interest and personal development, b) wanting to be able to help friends and family with minor aches and pains,c) giving massages as a side job, d) adding valuable skills to you own profession and e) seeking a career as a massage therapist.

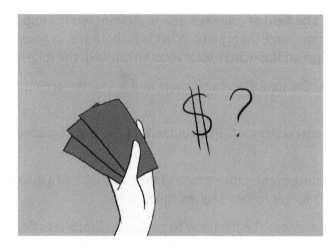

2. Set up a budget. It may not make sense for you to attend a 3-year massage course for a lot of money if you are only learning so that you can massage your spouse.

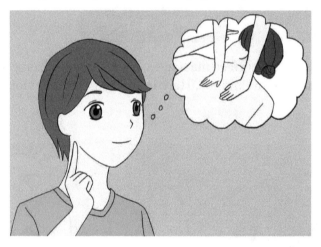

3. Determine which massage style you would like to learn: Decide whether you want to learn a hard massage style like Deep Tissue Massage or Rolfing or softer massage techniques such as Ayurvedic massage or lymph drainage, massage with accessories like hot stones, etc. Check books, magazines or on the Internet to learn about the major differences between these massage techniques.

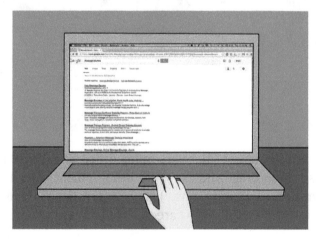

4. Shop around: Check on the Internet, yellow pages and local newspapers for massage courses being offered in your area.

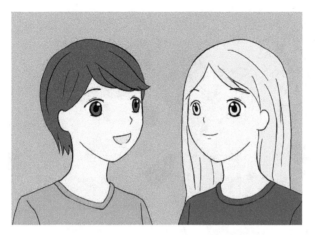

5. Ask around: Ask friends, family or colleagues if they know of any good massage courses in your area. Ask your local massage therapist where they learned massage.

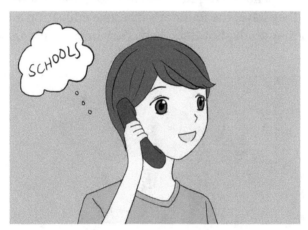

6. Contact different massage schools: Find out in advance about the contents of the course, their pricing and any other requirements for attending the course.

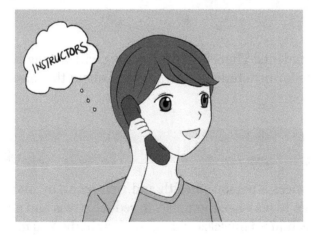

7. Contact the massage instructors: Speak to the instructors to see if the course is the right thing

for you and what teaching method they use. Ask what the ratio of theory to practice usually is in the course.

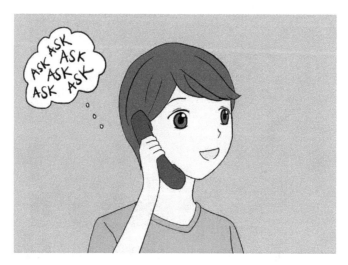

8. Check the credibility of the schools: Inquire as to how long the school has been in business, how many graduated students they have, the founder's massage education and the qualifications of the instructors (how long did they study, how long have they been teaching, what is their educational background, etc.).

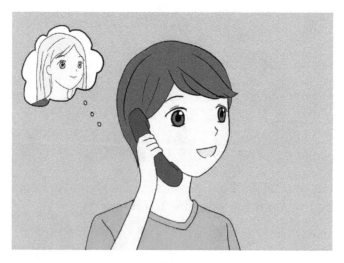

9. Try to contact former students: There is nothing wrong with asking for references. Ask some of the school's or instructor's former students how they feel about the massage course.

How to Start a Massage Therapy Business

A massage therapist enhances a person's health and well-being by manually manipulating their soft body tissues. People go to massage therapists to reduce stress and anxiety, to relax their muscles and to rehabilitate any injured muscles or areas of their body. You may be a practicing massage therapist who is ready to branch out on your own or you may be new to the profession and looking to start your own business. Though starting your own business as a massage therapist can be a big step, many massage therapists work for themselves, as it allows you to have a flexible work schedule and to maximize your profits.

Part 1. Getting the Necessary Certifications and Licenses

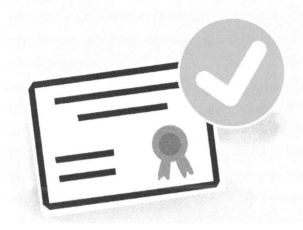

1. Complete your massage therapy certification. Before you can start a massage therapy business, you will need to complete massage therapy training and receive a certification as proof you have completed the necessary courses. A certification in massage therapy practice is considered an entry level qualification in the massage industry. You can receive certification through the National Certification Board for Therapeutic Massage and Bodywork (NCBTMB).

- There are many different types of massage therapy you can focus on and specialize in, such as remedial massage therapy or sports massage therapy. Though you may decide to specialize, you should be certified in extensive training on the essential techniques of massage, and have practicum hours at a clinic to get hands on experience.

- Most states in the U.S. require certification and licensing in order to register as a certified massage therapist. Alaska, Kansas, Montana, Oklahoma, and Wyoming are the only states that do not regulate massage therapists.

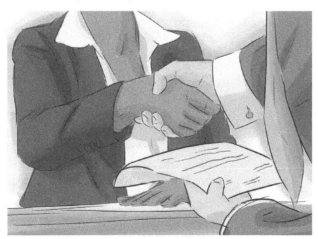

2. Apply for a business license: You should check with your local state laws on business registra-

tion to determine if you need a business license. Some states require you to obtain a business license if you sell massage therapy products in addition to massage therapy services. As a certified practitioner, you may also be required to obtain an "Art of Healing" license. You can find more information on business licenses by talking to the State Department of Revenue and Consumer Affairs, the county clerk, city hall, or the regulatory agency for massage therapy in your state or province.

- Reach out to your local small business association for more detailed information on the licensing laws required in your state or area, as they can often tell you exactly what is required for your type of business.

- The Associated Bodywork Massage Professionals (ABMP) gives its members access to information about the licensing requirements by state.

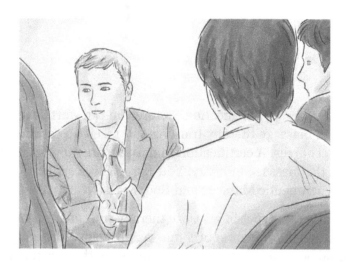

3. Join a massage therapy association: Massage therapy associations are a good way to network with other therapist and business owners. They also often offer benefits for their members like business advice, information on certification and licensing, and other opportunities. Some associations require members to pay to join, like the Associated Bodywork Massage Professionals (AMBP), and others have no membership fees.

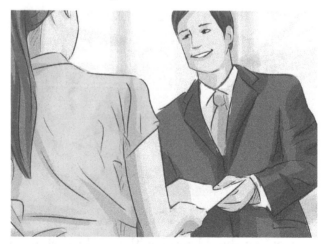

4. Get liability insurance: As the owner of a massage therapy business, you will be responsible for covering any liabilities from your clients. You will be working intensely and intimately with your clients so it is important that you protect yourself in the event you are sued by a client or have to claim damages or issues on your insurance. Getting liability insurance ensures you are protected and can afford to fight off a suit in court.

- As well, as a self-employed individual, you will need to provide your own health insurance coverage. You may also want to invest in disability insurance, which will protect you in the event you are injured and cannot work.

Part 2. Creating a Business Plan

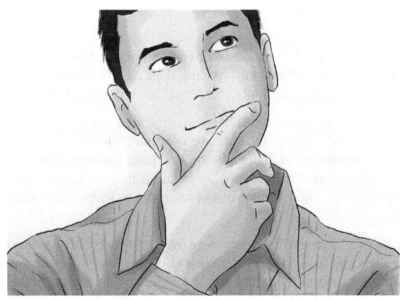

1. Choose your business name: Once you have sorted out the necessary certification and licensing, you will need to determine your business name. Your business name will act as branding, as it will be printed on your business cards and it will be clearly stated on your website and your social media accounts. Come up with at least two to three options for business names in the event one name is already taken by an existing business.

- You may want to use your given name as your business name, given it is an uncommon or unique name. It's likely the name "Massage by Carol Lumbort" will not be taken if you live in a small town or area, but a name like "Massage by Carol" could already be taken.

- Try to choose a business name that is unique to you but also easy to remember and read. You may decide to focus on a theme or idea that relates to massage therapy, such as "relaxation" "calming" "rehabilitation" or "releasing". To avoid overlapping with an existing business name, you may want to then personalize this theme so it is singular to you. For example, "Relaxation with Carol Lumbort" or "Lumbort's Calming Massage".

- You can confirm if your business name idea has already been trademarked by searching the United States Patent and Trademark Office database.

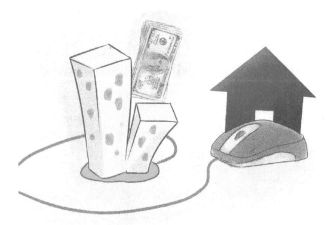

2. Decide if you are going to work from home or from an office: Many massage therapists work from their home and do home visits when servicing their clients. However, you may decide that you want to establish a separate office space where you can serve clients on site.

- Working from home means you will have less start up costs and very little overhead costs, as the majority of the profit will be going to you, not your rent or building maintenance. However, you will need to do many jobs at once, from booking clients to stocking supplies to bringing your massage therapy supplies to and from your clients' homes. You will likely need to also establish a home office in a spare room to keep your business documents organized.

- Renting or leasing a space will require more overhead costs and start-up costs. However, it would also allow you to service more clients at once and possibly turn a larger profit than just working on your own. You may decide to take on a business partner so you can combine your client list or hire other therapists to work in the location.

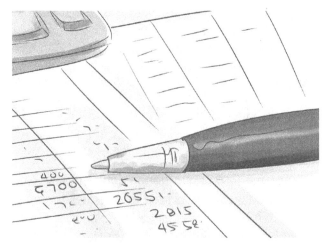

3. Outline your start-up expenses. Your business plan should have enough capital or start-up funds to cover several major expenses:

- Occupancy expenses: If you are renting or leasing a space, you will need to budget for your monthly rent and building maintenance costs. You will also need to consider other bills like a phone line, an internet connection, electricity, and heating. If you are using a home office, you may still need to budget for a separate phone line for your business.

- Operating expenses: These are expenses that are required during the day to day operation of your business. You may have operating expenses in the form of a web designer or graphic designer you hire for marketing, an accountant to file your taxes, or a massage therapist professional on contract to help you with your new practice. You may also have operating expenses in the form of materials, such as a ledger for your finances and massage therapy materials like lotions, creams, towels, blankets, and other massage supplies. You should list every possible operations item you can think of, even if it does not come into play later, to ensure you can cover everything in your budget.

- One-time expenses: These are considered "capital" expenses, which you only buy once as an investment in your business. If you have an office space, this may be furniture for the reception area and the massage room, or a computer for booking clients. If you work from home, you may decide to invest in electronic equipment that you will use primarily for your business. You will also need to invest in massage chairs for your office space or a portable massage chair you carry with you to your clients' homes.

- Marketing expenses: This could be the web designer fee for your business website, the graphic designer fee for designing your brochures and business cards, or other advertising that you invest in to generate business. Marketing is an essential tool for building your clientele and staying profitable as a small business.

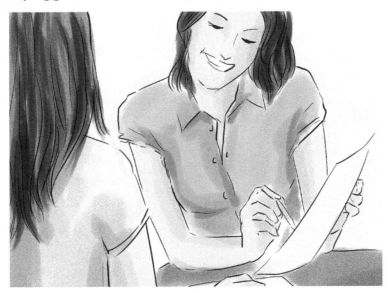

4. Apply for a business loan, if necessary: Once you have drawn up your business plan and considered all of your expenses, you should have a good sense of the start-up capital you require to get your business off the ground. You may then use this as a baseline against your own funds, the funds of an investor, or to apply for a small business loan from your bank.

- Many banks will require a business plan and other financial documents to consider you for a business loan. If you do not qualify for a business loan from your bank, you may want to apply at other banks.

- You may also want to consider talking to investors who may be interested in investing in your business. Use your business plan to convince them that your business is viable and a worthwhile investment for them.

Part 3. Finding and Retaining Clientele

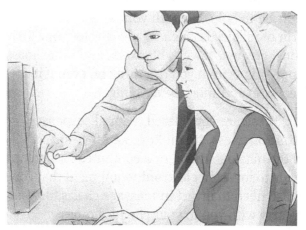

1. Create a website for your business: Many massage therapists use their website as a way to communicate with clients, book clients, and retain new clientele. The website does not have to be fancy or state of the art. Instead, go for a basic website that showcases your business name, your certifications, the services you offer, and your unique approach to massage therapy.

- You can hire a web designer to create your website for you, or create your own website using a basic website design program like Wordpress.com or Squarespace.com.

- You can then link your website to other social media accounts like Facebook, Instagram, and Twitter. Your business should also have a Google Plus page with accurate information that appears when your business is googled by clients.

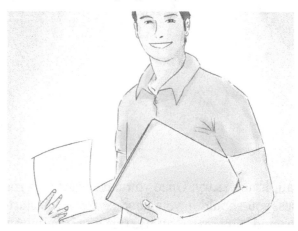

2. Hand out flyers in your community: Though it may seem old-fashioned to hand out flyers, targeting your community with old-fashioned marketing can be beneficial. Go around to local coffee shops and community centers and ask if you can post flyers about your new massage therapist business. This will help you develop business in your area and lead to word of mouth marketing.

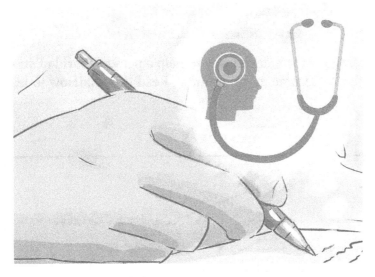

3. Register your business with health funds in your country: Some of your clients may want to claim their massage with their company's health fund or the government health fund so they can receive a rebate. You will need to make this option available to your clients by contacting each health fund and filling out an application form. You will then receive a provider number that you can use on your clients' rebates to allow them to claim their massages.

- Offering this option to your clients will likely make your business seem more appealing to clients and keep them coming back to you for your services.

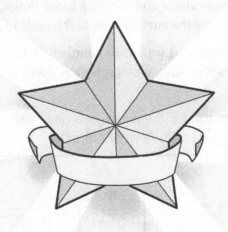

4. Reward referrals from existing clients: To encourage your clients to continue to use your services, you can start a rewards program where your clients get discounts or bonus treatments once they have booked you a certain number of times or spent a certain amount of money. You can also set up a referrals program where clients are rewarded if they refer a friend to your business.

- Using rewards programs can be a simple and direct way to retain your clients and to attract new clients. However, you should not lean too heavily on these programs, as your massage therapy services should be strong enough to justify return visits from your clients.

How to Give a Full Body Massage

Giving a full body massage is a wonderful way to help a person get rid of stress and sore muscles. It can also help two people become more intimate. Read this wikiHow to learn how to give a full body massage.

Part 1. Creating a Relaxing Atmosphere

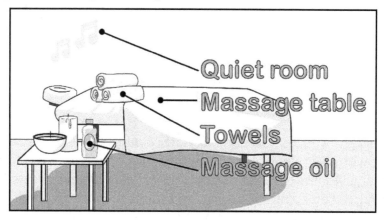

1. Make sure the room is comfortable: It is essential that the room is comfortable for conducting your massage. If your partner/client feels uncomfortable throughout the massage, they will not enjoy it as much.

- Make sure they have somewhere comfortable to lie down, such as a bed, a soft rug or a proper massage table. Cover the surface with soft towels to keep them clean and free of oil.

- Make sure the room is nice and warm. Remember that your partner/client will be partly undressed for the duration of the massage, so you don't want them to be cold. Use a space heater if necessary.

- Make sure the room you use for the massage is somewhere private where you will not be disturbed by any other people, children or animals.

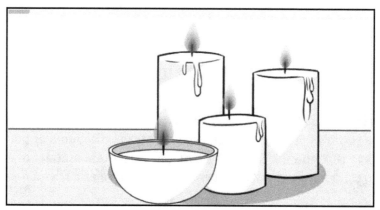

2. Light some candles: There's something very relaxing about candles, so it's a good idea to light a couple around the room.

- If possible, turn the lights down low or off completely and work only by candlelight. You want the person receiving the massage to be so relaxed that they're almost asleep by the end, so the darker it is the better.

- Use candles with relaxing (but not overpowering) scents, such as lavender or sea breeze, to contribute to the overall experience.

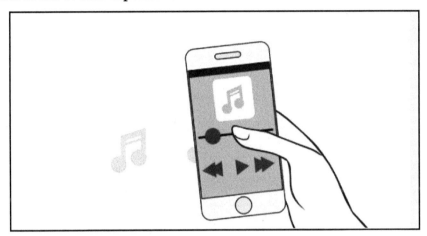

3. Play soothing music: Playing some soothing music can contribute to the calm and relaxing atmosphere of the massage. Gentle classical music, or sounds from nature are both good options.

- If possible, try to find out what type of music your partner/client enjoys. Remember that the massage is about them, not you, so you should try to cater to their tastes.

- Don't play the music too loud, it should be playing very softly in the background. It should add to the experience, not take away from it.

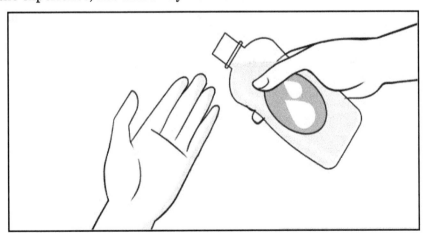

4. Use a massage oil: It is essential to use oil when giving a massage. It helps your hands to glide easily over the skin, so you don't cause pulling, pinching or any kind of pain to your partner/client.

- There are plenty of fancy (and expensive) store bought oils available, but any kind of natural oil will do just fine. For example, if you have sunflower or grape seed oil in your kitchen, you can use them for your massage. Jojoba and almond oils are also very effective and have a pleasant aroma.

- You can add a few drops of essential oil to your massage oil. You should use pure (natural and unadulterated) essential oils, not chemical perfume oils. Be aware that essential oils can penetrate the bloodstream, so choose wisely: opt for relatively gentle oils like lavender or orange. However, you should consult a medical professional first if your partner/client is pregnant or has any serious medical conditions.

- Try to warm the oil and your hands slightly before applying the oil to your partner/client's skin. Cold oil/hands are not conducive to a relaxing massage.

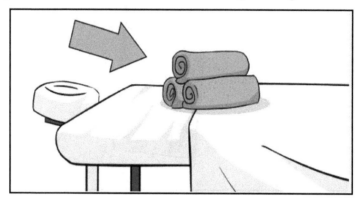

5. Have plenty of towels on hand: Make sure you have plenty of fresh, clean towels on hand for use during the massage.

- First you will need to cover the surface you are working on with towels in order to protect them from the massage oil (which can stain).

- Secondly, you will need towels to cover the your partner/client's body as you work on them. Ideally they should be stripped down to their underwear to leave as much skin exposed as possible. Then you can cover them with a towel to protect their modesty and to keep them warm while you are working on each body part.

- Thirdly, you will need extra towels to wipe the excess oil off you hands during and after the massage.

Part 2. Getting the Right Technique

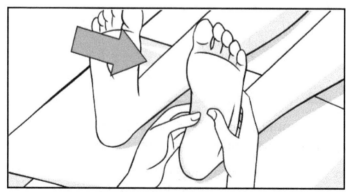

1. Begin with the feet: Start massaging the soles of the feet by wrapping both hands around the foot and using your thumbs to apply pressure.

- Pay special attention to the arch of each foot, as this area tends to accumulate a lot of tension, but also massage the heel and the ball of the foot.

- When you get to the toes, grab each one individually and give it a gentle pull, this helps to release any tension.

- Be aware that not everyone likes having their feet touched, and some people are very ticklish, so ask your partner/client before you touch their feet.

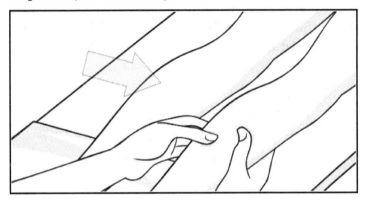

2. Work your way up the legs: When you're done with the feet, move onto the back of the legs. Give each leg a couple of long, relaxing strokes to begin with, all the way from the calf to the upper thigh.

- Apply light pressure with both hands, smoothly stretching the skin. This technique is known as effleurage, and is a good way to ease into the massage.

- Then, cover the leg you're not currently working on with a towel and focus on massaging the calf of one leg. Use a kneading technique (like kneading bread) to work the calf muscle.

- Move up towards the thigh and repeat the kneading technique here. Then press the heel of your hand into the skin and very slowly move it along the thigh. You should always move in the direction of the heart.

- Cover the leg you just finished working on with a towel (to keep in heat) and repeat the massage on the other leg.

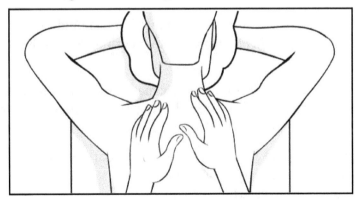

3. Move from the lower to the upper back. Use the effleurage technique described above to perform long, soft strokes, going from the top of the glutes to the base of the neck.

- Place the palm of each hand on either side of the spine and work your way up, keeping your hands parallel to one another. When you reach the top of the back, fan your hands outwards across the shoulders, as if outlining the top of a heart.

- Return to the lower back and use a kneading motion to work the large muscles on either side of the spine. These areas tend to build up a lot of tension, so make sure to spend some time here.

- Next, use a "press and release" technique to work your way up the back. This involves pressing your fingertips firmly into the flesh of the back before quickly releasing. When the pressure is released, your partner/client's brain will release a rush of pleasurable chemicals.

- When you get to the upper back, have your partner/client bend their elbows so their shoulder blades stick out. This will give you better access to the muscle around the edge of the shoulder blades, which tends to harbor a lot of tension and knots.

- To work on the knots, use a thumb or single finger to press and release repeatedly around the problem area.

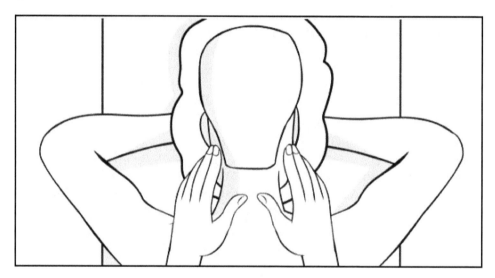

4. Do the neck and shoulders. When you've finished with the shoulders, use the press and release technique to massage along the neck, all the way to the hairline. Remember to keep your hands on either side of the spine.

- Place a hand on either shoulder in the classic massage position and knead the thumbs deep into the muscles of the shoulders. Use your fingers for grip, but don't press them into the collarbone, as this can be painful.

- Now move around to stand in front of your client/partner's head, so their shoulders are facing you. Make a fist with each hand, then rub the knuckles gently but firmly across the tops of the shoulders, to release any tension,

- Next use your thumbs to press and release along the tops of the shoulders and up the back of the neck.

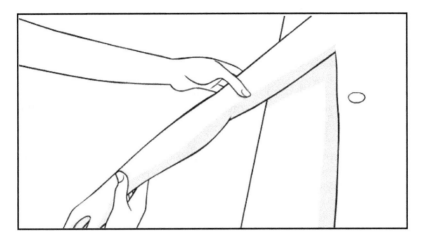

5. Massage the hands and arms. When you're done with the neck and shoulders, move onto the arms, working on one at a time.

- Hold your partner/client's wrist in your left hand, so their entire arm is lifted from the bed. Then use your right hand to sweep along the back of the forearm, along the tricep and over the shoulder, coming back on the opposite side.

- Now, switch to holding their wrist in your right hand, then sweep your left hand along their forearm and bicep, then over the shoulder and down the opposite side.

- Place your partner/client's arm back on the bed, the use your fingers and thumbs to gently knead the forearms and upper arms.

- To massage the hands, take their hand in yours and massage the palm with your thumbs, using small circular motions. Then, take each finger in turn and slowly slide from the knuckles to the nail. Pull each finger firmly, but not so hard that you cause it to crack!

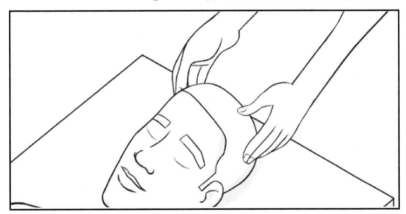

6. End with the head: Ask your client/partner to flip over so you can work on the head and face. Give them a moment if they need to rearrange their towel.

- Use your thumbs to gently massage the top of the scalp. For added pleasure, use your nails to scratch slightly.

- Next, massage the folds and lobe of each ear between your thumb and forefinger. Then use your fingertips to gently swipe along the contours of the cheekbones and not.

- Put your hands beneath your partner/client's head and lift it slightly from the bed. Use your fingers to find the small hollows when the neck meets the base of the skull. Apply firm pressure with your fingertips, then release. Repeat several times.

- Put your hands underneath the jaw and pull the head gently upwards, to stretch the neck muscles. Now, gently press the center of the forehead (between the eyebrows) with your fingertips and release. Repeat for 30 seconds.

- Next use your fingertips to gently massage the temples, moving in slow circular motions. The temples are an important acupressure point, so this helps to relieve tension.

Part 3. Perfecting the Massage

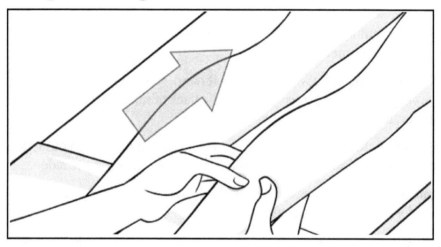

1. Work slowly: Never try to rush through the massage - it should be a luxurious, relaxing experience for your partner/client.

- Dedicate time to each individual body part, giving it your full care and attention, and keep your strokes long, smooth and slow.

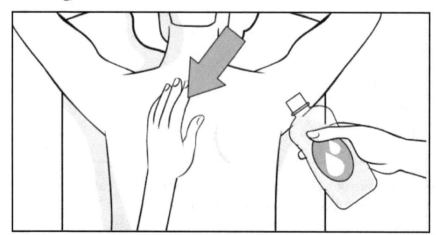

2. Keep your hands in contact with the skin at all times. Your hands should be in contact with your client/partner's skin for the full duration of the massage - this keeps the momentum flowing and never breaks the atmosphere of relaxation.

- Even if you have to grab a towel, a drink of water or more massage oil during the massage, try to keep one hand on the skin at all times.

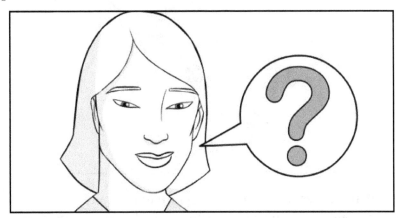

3. Communicate: Communication is key throughout a massage. What feels good to you mightn't feel good to the other person, so it's important to ask them how they're feeling and to really take on board their responses.

- Ask them how the pressure feels, where they would like you to work on and what they enjoy the most. However, try to speak in a low, soothing voice to maintain the calm atmosphere.

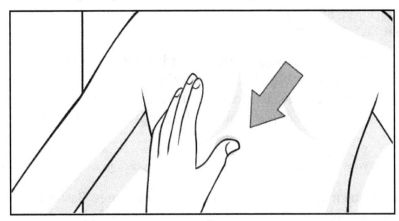

4. Pay attention to knots: If the person you're working on has a lot of knots in their back, it's a good idea to work on them to try to release them.

- However, make sure to ask your partner or client first, as some people find this too painful and would rather not ruin their relaxing massage.

- The knots may feel like large, circular areas of tightness, or tiny bumps which almost feel like peas beneath the skin. Try to get directly on top of the knot, otherwise it can slip out from beneath your fingers.

- Apply increasing pressure to the knot, then rotate your thumb or finger to try to undo it. You may need to rotate in opposite directions in order to work it out fully.

- Try not to get too involved in any deep tissue work though - this is best left to qualified massage therapists. Stick to what feels good for you partner/client.

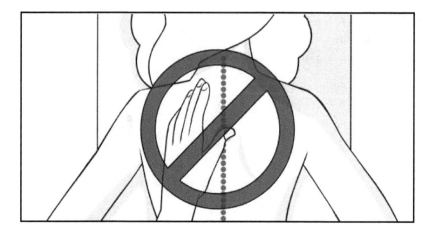

5. Avoid the spine and any bones: Never apply pressure to the spine or any other bones. This will feel unpleasant and uncomfortable for your partner/client and has the potential to cause more harm than good.

- Besides, it is the muscles you really need to work on, as this is where the most tension collects. Stick to the muscles and you can't go wrong.

Hot Stone Massage

Hot stone massage is a type of massage therapy that involves the use of smooth, heated stones. The massage therapist places the hot stones on specific points on your body and may also hold the stones while giving the massage. The localized heat and weight of the stones warm and relax muscles, allowing the massage therapist to apply deeper pressure to those areas without causing discomfort.

How does Hot Stone Massage Differ from other Types of Massage

The hallmark of hot stone massage is the use of the heated stones. Basalt river rocks are typically used because they are smooth (from the river's current) and retain heat well.

In preparation for the treatment, the massage therapist heats the stones in a professional stone heater until they are within a precise temperature range, typically between 110 and 130 degrees Fahrenheit. (Stones that are too hot can cause burns.)

While massage therapists often use anatomy to guide the placement of the stones, some therapists will also place stones on points thought to energetically balance the mind and body.

Swedish massage therapy techniques are typically used during the massage, which may include long strokes and kneading and rolling.

Benefits

People often describe hot stone massage as comforting and deeply relaxing. The warmth is soothing for people who tend to feel chilly.

The heat of the stones relaxes muscles, allowing the therapist to work deeper while using lighter pressure.

There is a lack of research on the benefits of hot stone massage. People often use hot stone massage for the following conditions:

- Anxiety
- Back pain
- Depression
- Insomnia

Is it Painful

The hot stones are smooth and typically several inches long. The stones should be warmed using a professional electric massage stone heater so that the temperature can be controlled. If the stones are too hot or uncomfortable, be sure to let the massage therapist know immediately. Stones that are too hot can cause burns.

The heat of the stones allows the massage therapist work on deep tissue, if needed. As with any massage, however, massage therapy shouldn't hurt and you should tell your massage therapist if you feel any pain.

What to Expect

During the massage, the therapist places stones on specific points on the body. While the points may vary depending on the areas of muscle tension and the client's health history, the stones are generally placed in the following areas:

- Along both sides of the spine
- In the palms of your hand
- On your legs, abdomen, feet

Small stones may be placed between the toes or on the forehead.

After the stones are placed on your body, it may take a few minutes for the heat to penetrate the sheet or towel so you can discern whether the stones are too hot.

The therapist applies massage oil to the skin. Holding stones in both hands, the therapist uses gliding movements to move the stones along the muscles. The therapist uses Swedish massage techniques on the back, legs, neck, and shoulders while the stones are in place or after they have been removed.

The length of a typical hot stone massage is between 60 and 90 minutes.

Who Shouldn't Get a Hot Stone Massage

While hot stone massage is generally considered safe when performed by a trained and licensed massage therapist, it's not right for everyone. Consult your doctor if you have a medical condition, such as high blood pressure, diabetes, heart disease, varicose veins, migraines, autoimmune disease, decreased pain sensitivity, cancer, autoimmune disease, epilepsy, tumors, or metal implants, or are on medication that thins the blood.

Also, check with your doctor if you have had recent surgery or have recent wounds or areas of weakened or inflamed skin.

Pregnant women and children should avoid hot stone massage.

To prevent burns, a professional massage stone heater should be used (microwaves, ovens, hot plates, and slow cookers should never be used).

Final Thoughts

Hot stone massage has continued to evolve, with many massage therapists and spas offering their own versions of the massage.

Whether you're trying massage for the first time or are already a fan and interested in trying something new, talk with your massage therapist (and healthcare provider) about whether hot stone massage is appropriate for you. While many people find the warmth deeply relaxing and beneficial for the mind, body, and spirit, you also want to make sure that it's right type of bodywork for you—especially if you have a health condition or injury.

Some additional tips on making the most out of your massage:

- Don't eat before your massage.
- Stay hydrated by drinking water before and after your massage.
- Let your therapist know if the stones are too warm or the pressure too intense.
- See a licensed massage therapist trained in hot stone massage.
- Be thorough when completing the intake form.

How to do Hot Stone Massage

Hot stone massage uses a combination of warmed stones and massage techniques to relax tense muscles, relieve pain and stiffness, and improve circulation. The treatment can be used for ailments like muscular aches, arthritic conditions, and autoimmune disorders. The heat of the stones penetrates the skin to promote better blood flow, release toxins and create a deeper muscle relaxation than in a standard massage. By placing the warmed stones over acupressure points you can help release the flow of energy and promote the body's own healing process. Those who do hot stone massage can also customize the treatment to a client's specific needs and preferences. It is vitally important that you use caution and pay close attention to your participant. Burns from hot stones are the #1 reason for lawsuits against licensed massage therapists.

Part 1. Gathering your Materials

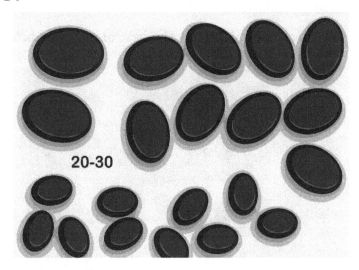

1. Find or purchase stones: Stones used in this treatment are typically made of basalt, due to their ability to retain heat. The stones should also be very smooth, so they do not irritate the skin in any way. If you can't find basalt stones, however, smooth river rocks are fine.You can order a hot stone massage kit online from Amazon or eBay. Do not want buy your stones from a rock quarry unless you are able to choose each stone individually.

- You should have anywhere between 20-30 stones, though some professional massages may have upwards of 45-60. There should be at least two large ovals around 8" long to 6" wide, seven stones you can fit in the palm of your hand, and 8 small stones between the size of an egg or a quarter.

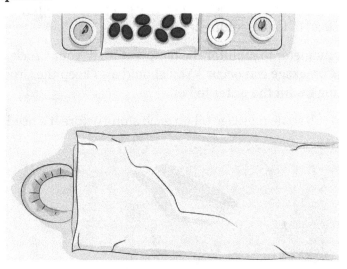

2. Set up your area: If you do not have a massage table, a bed or the floor will be fine. Once you've chosen where the massage should take place, you should lay out a clean sheet or a thick towel for the person you are massaging to lay down on. This will not only help them be more comfortable but also help absorb any excess oil from the massage.

- To really create a relaxing environment, try lighting some aromatherapy candles. Soothing scents like lavender, lemongrass, eucalyptus, and vanilla will help immerse your participant in the massage experience.

- You can also try playing some quiet classical music, or rain sounds to add to the mood.

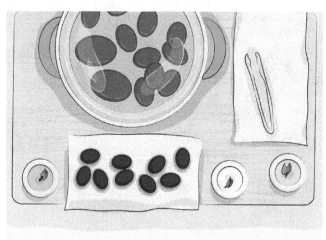

3. Heat up your stones: Ideally, you should prepare your stones 30-60 minutes before you begin your massage. The water should be no more than 130°. The stones will cool down as you use them. Anything below 110° is considered a warm stone massage, although it is important to know that a 104° stone can still burn someone if it is left laying on bare skin for a few minutes.

- To heat the stones, use a Crock-Pot that can hold at least 6 quarts of water or a large tabletop skillet that has sides close to 3 inches (7.6 cm). Note that Crock-Pots and similar kitchen equipment heat on a cycled basis, which means that the temperature can vary and must be monitored closely. It is better i f you can find something with an actual temperature setting, instead of low-medium-high.

- Use a meat thermometer to monitor the temperature in your Crock-pot. (Never use a glass thermometer as breakage can occur.) You should also keep the Crock-pot setting to warm or low, as you don't want the water to boil.

- You should also rub some massage oil on each stone before it's used.

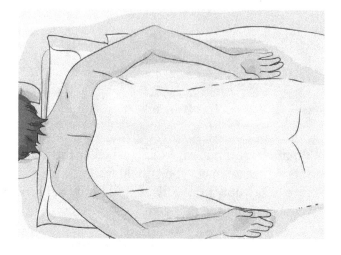

4. Never place a hot stone directly on the participant's skin without moving it. The pictures you see in spa advertisements are not accurate, they are just meant to look appealing. To prevent burns, you must place a flannel sheet or towel down and then put the stones on top of that.

- Keep in mind it can take 3-4 minutes for the heat of the stones to penetrate to the skin.

Part 2. Performing the Massage

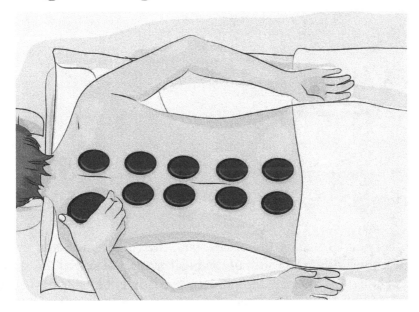

1. Please note that you should never have a participant lay down on top of hot stones as serious burns can occur.

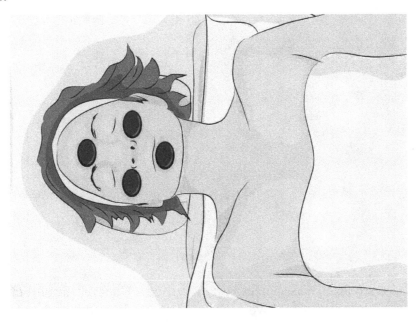

2. Place four small sized stones on the participant's face: Once the participant has settled, take four of the smaller stones, without oil, and place them on the acupressure areas on their face. There should be one stone on their forehead, one under their lips, and one on each of their cheeks. You

should avoid putting oil on these stones as it may clog their pores or irritate their skin. A great alternative is to chill the stones for the face instead of heating them as this will help reduce any puffiness.

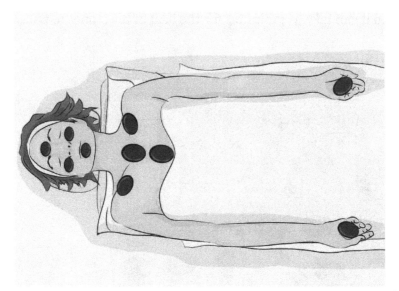

3. Put medium to large stones along the breastbone, the collarbones, and in the participant's hands. Depending on the height and width of the participant, the size of the stones you use may vary. However, you should try to place one stone or more on either side of their collarbone, two large ones along the breastbone, and two palm-sized stones in their hands. They do not need to clasp these, but should instead remain fully relaxed and gently cupping the stones.

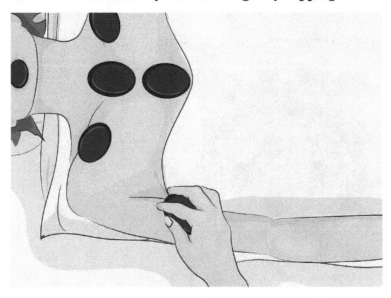

4. Use two palm-sized stones to massage the rest of the body: Uncover the part of the body you are going to massage, remembering to remove any placed stones first. Rub some oil onto the skin and the stones. Follow the cords of muscles to work out any knots, changing stones as needed as they cool. When finished, re-cover the area you massaged, replace any stones and move on to the next area. Remove all stones once you have completed the entire massage.

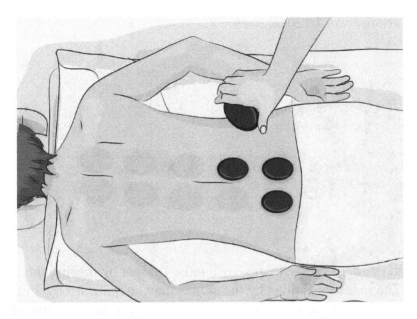

5. Turn the participant over: After you've finished massaging the front, have the participant turn over to lie on their stomach.To make the participant more comfortable, try placing a rolled up towel under their ankles.

- You should also make sure that you are changing your stones so they stay warm.

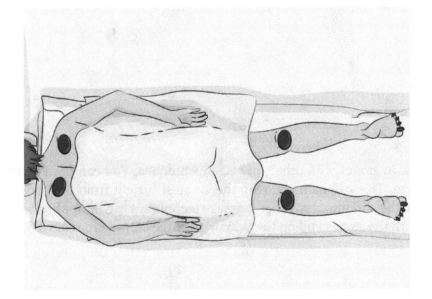

6. Cover the participant and place stones on the shoulder blades, the backs of the kneecaps, and between the toes. Pick larger stones for the shoulder blades and the backs of the kneecaps. For the toes, place a small stone between each. You should then wrap each foot in a towel to help hold in the warmth and keep the stones in place.

- After you've placed these, uncover the area you intend to massage and rub some oil into the the skin. take two palm-sized, oiled stones and use them to massage the participant. As before, re-cover the area massaged, replace any stones and move on to the next area.

Part 3. Trying Different Techniques

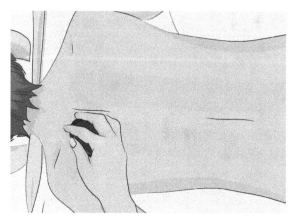

1. Use the stones to massage rather than your hands: Do this by moving the stones gently over tense, sore areas. The pressure applied by the stones may be quite strong, but since the participant's muscles have been sufficiently relaxed by the heating process, the procedure should virtually be painless.

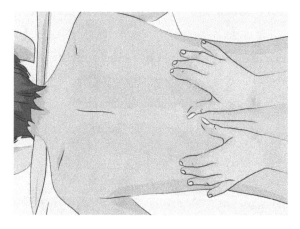

2. Combine the warm stones with other massage techniques: You can try a Swedish massage or deep tissue massage. This will help you reap the greatest benefit from the experience. While the stones heat and soothe stiff muscles, other massage techniques can be applied with little or no discomfort - either with the stones still on the skin or after the stones are removed.

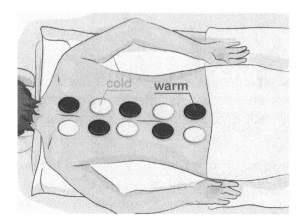

3. Alternate the hot stones with cold marble stones: Most clients find that after a period of time, their bodies become so relaxed from the hot stone massage techniques, they don't even notice the temperature change to the cooler stones. This process is often recommended for soothing injuries that result in painful swelling or inflammation.

How to Give a Leg Massage

Giving someone a leg massage can be a way to help relieve leg pain caused by things like overexertion. Help the person find a comfortable position and then work your way from the feet upward. If leg pain is persistent, it may be caused by an underlying health condition. If someone's leg pain does not pass on its own, they should see a doctor.

Part 1. Establishing the Basics

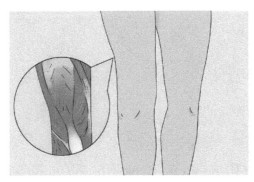

1. Learn about basic anatomy: It's helpful to know some anatomy before you give a massage. Thigh muscles are in 4 basic groups which run from the hips down to the knee, in the front, sides, and backs of the legs. Knowing where the bones are located should also be helpful because the tissues that connect muscle to bone are important to massage.

- The connective tissues around the joints, like the hips, the knees, the ankles and the feet, can be pulled, kneaded, or compressed.

- The hamstrings and calves in the back of the leg are notoriously tight and people who run often have issues related to the outer thigh area, the TFL, or the IT band.

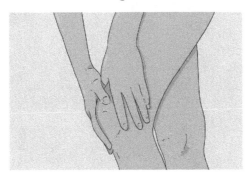

2. Figure out how to apply pressure: Start the massage with gentle techniques and use lighter pres-

sure near bones and sensitive areas. As circulation increases, so can the intensity of the massage. Move your fingers and hands quickly and lightly or slowly and firmly, but not quickly and firmly.

- The body parts you use to perform a massage affect the pressure. The elbows generally provide the strongest pressure. The palms and fingers will generally apply less pressure.

- Deeper tissue massage can include pressing down with the heel of the hand, the thumb, one hand on top of the other hand, the knuckles, a fist, or the forearm.

- Types of massage include gliding, kneading, compression, friction, percussion, vibration, jostling and range of motion movements.

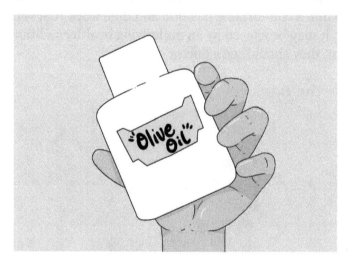

3. Choose your oils (optional): If you want, it's okay to use oil for a leg massage. This can make it easier to run your hands and fingers over someone's legs and oils can also provide a soothing effect. For leg massages, go for oils like olive oil, avocado oil, or almond oil. You can also use essential oils, or oils that are infused with scents such as lavender, eucalyptus, and tea tree, for a pleasantly aromatic experience.

- Make sure the person you're massaging does not have an existing allergy to the oil you use.

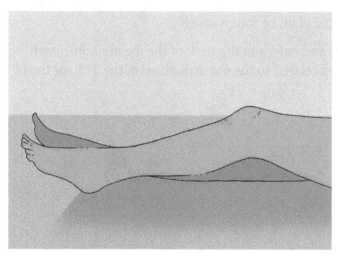

4. Find a comfortable position: To start, help the person you're massaging find a comfortable po-

sition. For leg massages, it's usually easy to lie down somewhere like a bed. The person can have their legs stretched forward. If you're only massaging one leg, you may want to have the person lie on their side with the leg you're massaging extending upward. You can also have the person lie with their legs stretched out and elevated slightly. A pillow can be used to elevate the person's legs.

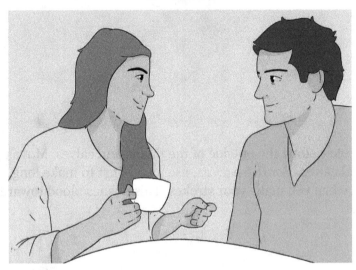

5. Communicate with the person: Ask the person if there's a particular area where they want extra pressure or attention. For example, if someone's thighs are bothering them, they may want you to focus on massaging their thighs. You may want to linger on certain areas and give them more attention.

Part 2. Massaging both Legs

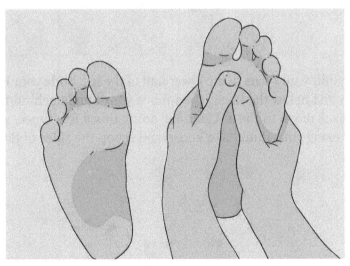

1. Start at the foot: Starting at the foot and stroking upward helps promote blood circulation, which can help ease pain and tension in the legs. Sandwich the person's foot between your palms. Then, put some oil into your palm and rub the foot firmly for a few minutes. When you're done rubbing the foot between your hands, give the foot a few gentle strokes moving from the toes to ankles.

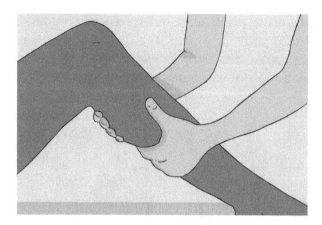

2. Use long, gentle strokes along the outside of the thighs and calves. Move upward from the foot towards the thighs and calves. For these areas, use a loose fist to make long, gentle strokes. Move from the foot upward when you make your strokes. This pushes blood towards the heart, increasing blood circulation.

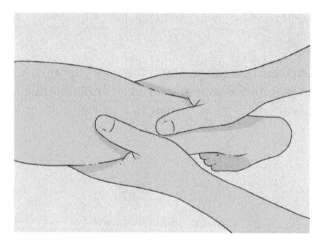

3. Massage the calves. Shift your focus to the lower half of the leg. Slide your hands up over the shin area from the ankle to just below the knee. Then move your hands behind the leg to the calf area and slide all the way back down to the ankle. After doing this a few times, work your way up and down the lower leg by using your thumbs to knead and scoop the sides of the leg.

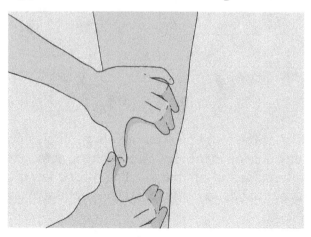

4. Finish by massaging the thighs: Work your way up the thigh area. Make scooping passes with your hands on the outside and inside of the leg to stimulate the different muscles in the upper leg. Apply some pressure as you use your palm to press near the center of the upper thigh and gluteal areas.

Part 3. Taking Safety Precautions

1. Be very gentle with swollen legs: If legs are swollen due to medical reasons, be very gentle. Make sure to check with the person to make sure they're comfortable. Use the lightest pressure possible when massaging swollen legs.

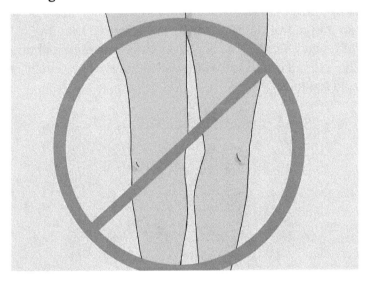

2. Avoid massaging the inner thighs on a pregnant woman: If you're massaging a pregnant woman's legs, stay away from massaging the inner thighs. Blood clots are more common in this area during pregnancy and massaging the area can dislodge clots. This can be a very serious, even fatal, problem.

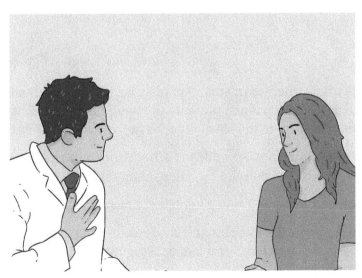

3. See a doctor for chronic leg pain. Leg pain can indicate health problems such as a leg injury or

chronic conditions like arthritis. While massages can temporarily relieve, frequent leg pain should be evaluated by a medical professional.

How to Release Carpal Tunnel Syndrome with Massage Therapy

Carpal tunnel syndrome is caused by a compression of the median nerve at the wrist and is associated with numbness, tingling, pain or a dull ache in the fingers, hand or wrist. If left untreated, it can cause severe pain and motor deficits, which can affect your ability to work and even cause temporary disability. Massage therapy can help treat and prevent carpal tunnel syndrome by promoting circulation, relieving inflammation, aiding in removal of metabolic residues, and soothing the irritated muscles and tendons.

Method 1. Massaging Therapy for Carpal Tunnel Syndrome

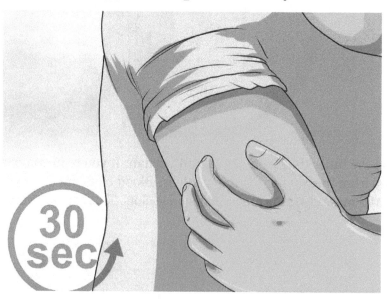

1. Apply light pressure to the muscles in your shoulder, arm, wrist and hand. Start your massage using light strokes and avoiding too much pressure (a technique called effleurage). Start from the shoulder and move down the arm to the small muscles in your wrist and fingers.

- Apply effleurage for at least 30 seconds to each section/muscle between your shoulder and hand. This will prepare the muscles for a deeper massage.

- Use the palm of your hand and your thumb and fingers to apply the massage.

- You can concentrate on the muscles and tendons on the wrist but because carpal tunnel syndrome is rarely strictly a wrist problem, massaging the muscles in the arm and shoulder area may also be beneficial.

- Optionally, you can use massage oil to reduce friction.

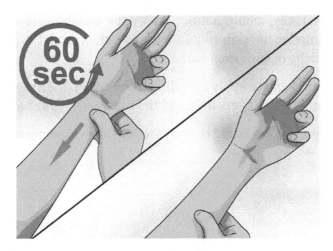

2. Apply deeper pressure friction massage to the shoulder, arm, wrist and hand. Friction technique accelerates the return flow of lymphatic and venous drainage and relieves edema. It also works in the treatment of scar tissues and adhesions.

- Apply deeper pressure using long, gliding strokes with your thumb.

- Start at the wrist area by pushing into the muscle in the center of the wrist, while gliding up to the elbow at the same time.

- Return back down the upper arm, into the elbow, forearm, and wrist.

- You can use your knuckles to provide more pressure without straining your hand. Apply enough pressure to feel the effect in the deep tissues but not so much that it causes severe pain.

- Also, massage your fingers and the palm of the hand by using light pressure and gentle stretches.

- Do at least 60 seconds of friction massage on each section/muscle, concentrating on the wrist but also working the knots and adhesions in the shoulder, arm and hand.

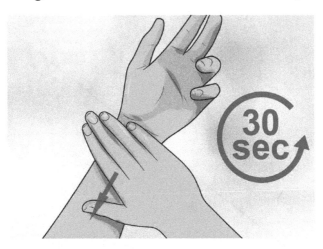

3. Apply kneading massage to the muscles in your shoulder, arm, wrist and hand. The kneading

technique, also called petrissage manipulation, causes the metabolic residues that have accumulated in the muscles and under the skin to join back into the circulation. Kneading may also improve the tonus and elasticity of your muscles.

- Use the palm of your hand to apply kneading technique to the muscles in your shoulder and arm, and your thumb and fingers to knead the muscles in your hand and wrist.

- Do at least 30 seconds of kneading to each section/muscle, concentrating on the wrist area.

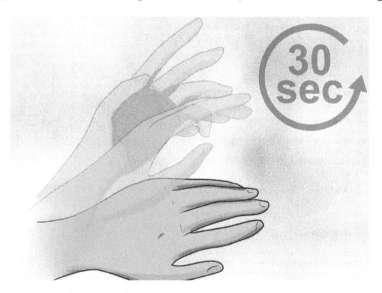

4. Apply shaking manipulation to the muscles in your shoulder, arm, wrist and hand. Shaking manipulation is shown to have a pain-relieving effect, while strengthening your atonic muscles. Extend your fingers and use the side of your hand to gently strike the muscles.

- You can also use the tips of your fingers or the heel to apply the technique.

- Do at least 30 seconds of shaking massage to each section/muscle, again concentrating on the wrist.

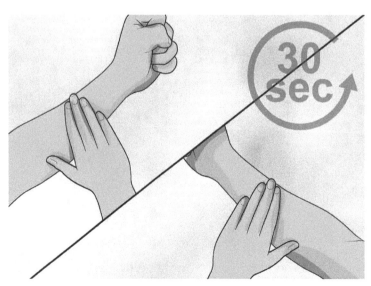

5. Apply effleurage to finish the massage: The massage should start and end with light massaging (or effleurage). Effleurage technique helps relax muscles and calms the nerves.

- Do at least 30 seconds of effleurage manipulation to each section/muscle to finish the series of massaging techniques.

- After you have completed one hand, repeat the massage to your other shoulder, arm, wrist and hand.

- The number of massaging sessions you need varies depending on the severity of the carpal tunnel syndrome. Sometimes you may see a relief in just one session, but often times you should see improvement between five and 10 sessions.

- If the symptoms persist or become worse, consult a doctor or a physical therapist.

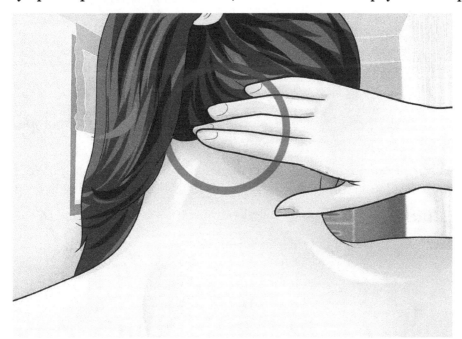

6. Apply acupressure to the muscle trigger points: Acupressure spots, or more commonly known as trigger points or muscle knots, can refer pain to the carpal tunnel area. These spots can also be found in the neck and shoulder area. To fully get any benefit, it's important to see a health professional that is trained in trigger point or acupressure treatments.

- Rest your forearm on a table, palm-up. Apply pressure to the muscles near the inside elbow — press down and see if this recreates your carpal tunnel pain. If it does, press gently for up to 30 seconds; the pain should gradually reduce.

- Move down the length of your forearm, testing for spots that recreate the carpal tunnel pain, then applying pressure for 30 seconds.

- Turn your arm so that it is palm-down and perform similar pressure on any tender spots you find between your elbow and wrist.

- Perform this exercise daily.

Method 2. Stretching Exercises for Carpal Tunnel Syndrome

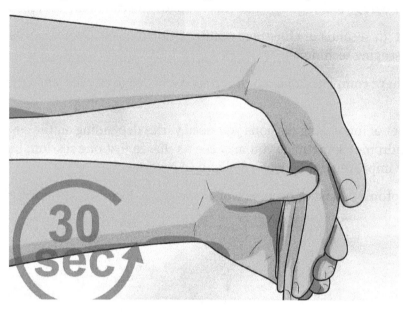

1. Stretch your wrist flexors and forearm: Hold your arm straight out in front of you, palm up, and bend your hand down so that your fingers point to the floor.

- Optionally, you can do this kneeling on the floor by placing the palms of your hands on the floor (fingers pointing toward you). Shift your body backward until you feel the stretch.

- Hold the stretch for at least 30 seconds.

- Repeat with the other hand.

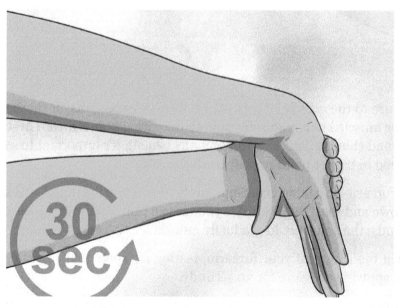

2. Stretch your wrist extensors and forearm: This is almost identical to the previous stretch except you will extend your arm with your palm downward this time. Bend your hand down so that your fingers point to the floor.

- Hold the stretch for at least 30 seconds.
- Repeat with the other hand.

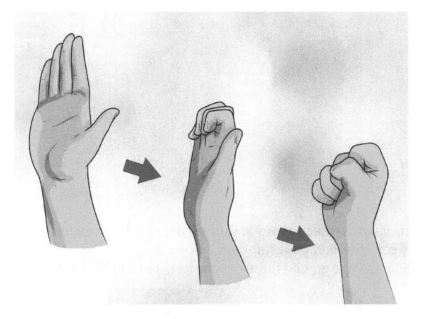

3. Perform tendon gliding stretches: This is a series of movements during which your fingers reach five positions: straight, hook, fist, tabletop, and straight fist.

- Start with the straight position by holding your fingers straight up and together.
- Bend your fingertips down to lightly touch the palm (if you can).
- Move your fingers to a partially closed fist.
- Bend your fingers straight forward with your thumb underneath (like forming a birds head).
- Finally, form a fully closed fist with your thumb relaxed on the side.
- Repeat this series of movements a few times with both hands.

How to Avoid Injury

Anyone who works intensively with their hands is prone to injuring their arms, wrists, thumbs, and fingers. Unfortunately, massage therapists are no exception. The arms and hands are just not designed to withstand heavy work over extended periods of time, and repetitive actions can easily lead to carpal tunnel syndrome, tennis elbow and other hand and wrist RSIs. It is rare for massage therapists to be taught how to protect their bodies and this leads to an exceptionally high rate of injury in the profession. Yet the good news is that it doesn't have to be this way. If you know the correct way to position and use your body and hands, you can have a long and healthy career. Protecting your hands is easy when you absorb the principles of dynamic body use; better yet, it also helps to give your clients an even better treatment.

Part 1. Proper Body Mechanics

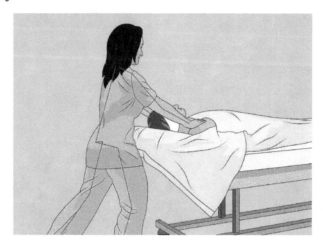

1. Use good body mechanics while you work; this will not only help you to avoid injury but enables you to use a more sensitive and powerful touch. Good body mechanics require having a strong energetic connection with the ground through your feet, legs and hara (belly).

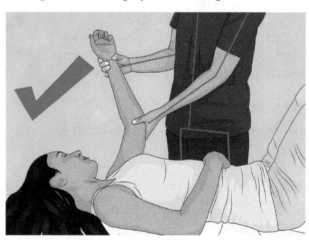

2. Point your stomach towards the subject of your work: Your hara should usually be pointed in the direction of your work. Imagine your hara as a strong light that shines where you are working.

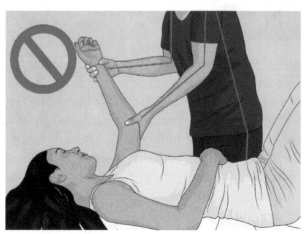

3. Do not bend: Never bend your back to carry out a move. Lunge forwards in a tai chi stance, or kneel down if necessary.

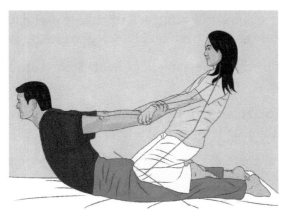

4. Use your body weight, not muscular strength, to work deeper. Always remember "lean don't press."

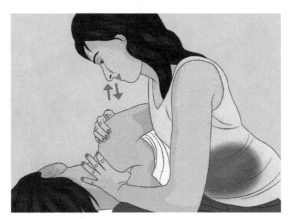

5. Breathe into your belly. Always find the quiet part within yourself by re-connecting with the breath.

Part 2. Massage stance

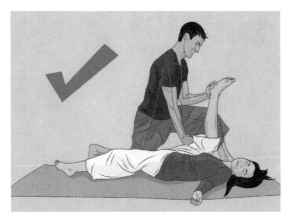

1. Choose a proper stance: While working, your body should mainly be in one of the four stances

described below. Using a massage stance should be a dynamic dance, allowing you to flow from one position to the other, depending on what is best for your body at that time.

- Forward Tai Chi stance: Similar to a lunge. Particularly useful for effleurage based strokes. Weight can transfer between the front and back leg to give power.

- Horse stance: Feet hip width apart and legs bent. Make sure knees roll outwards rather than medially to prevent strain.

- Kneeling Tai Chi stance: This can be used to maintain good body mechanics when you need to be at a lower level than standing would allow.

- Seated: Have legs wide apart and both feet firmly connected to the ground. Make sure that your own spine is not slumped.

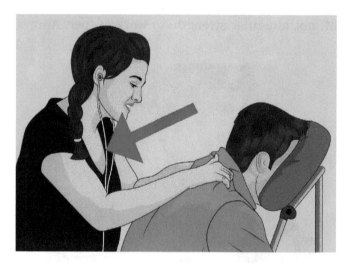

2. Take the opportunity to move and dance while you work. Put on some great music, move your hips, and enjoy yourself.

Part 3. Correct use of Breath

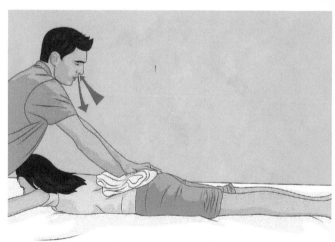

1. Use breath to remain calm: The breath is a great tool for helping you to calm down, ground yourself, and deepen your intention and pressure while working. Get into the habit of regularly checking into your breath and body while treating; you will find that at moments of stress, you will tend to hold your breath and tense up your whole body. Check into the "space between breaths", namely, the slight pause after you breathe out and before you breathe in, to remind yourself of the power of "less is more."

- You can deepen your pressure simply by breathing energy up from the earth through your legs and down your arms and hands.

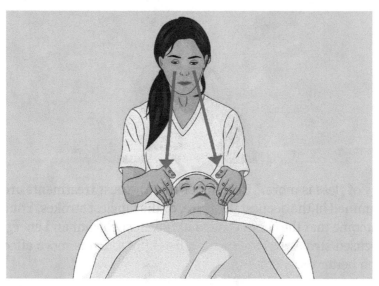

2. Use breath to focus: When you feel anxious or not good enough, take a few deep breaths into your belly – this will calm you and slow you down. Remind yourself you are good enough.

Part 4. Listening to your Body

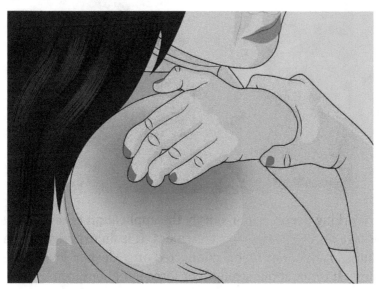

1. Learn to recognize strain: During treatments, use your breath to regularly check into your body. Scan yourself from head to foot to see if anything is feeling strained or tired. If you are hurt, change

what you are doing! Also, listen to your body between treatments. If you feel tired, in pain, weepy or irritable after a day's work, you need to change something about what you are doing – less massages per day, or longer gaps between treatments.

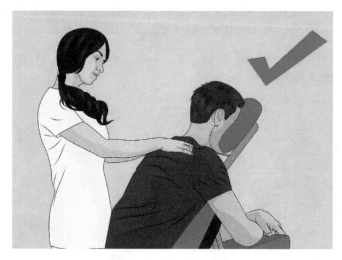

2. Use the principles of "less is more." Remember that the best treatments are not those with the most techniques crammed in,the deepest pressure, or the fanciest strokes. Your goal should always be to achieve the outcome that the client desires in the most elegant and energy efficient way. One thoughtful, slow, focused stroke executed with a listening touch is more effective than ten hasty ones. This feels much better too.

Part 5. Using Body Weight and Energy to Work Deeper

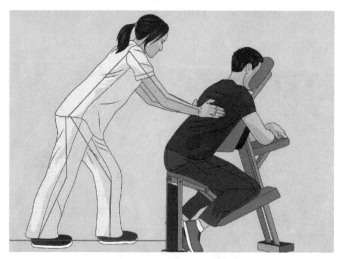

1. Engage properly: Working deeply is not simply the application of deep pressure to the body. It is not a 'harder' massage or a more rigorous treatment. It is an experience of engaging the body's tissue and its structures in a manner that is connected on a 'deeper' level. 'Deeper' in connection, contact, and awareness. It is not about strength or force but about focus.

- You are able to work deeper by using your body weight to lean into the tissues and having the intention and breath to penetrate deeper into the tissues.

Part 6. Using a Wide Variety of Techniques

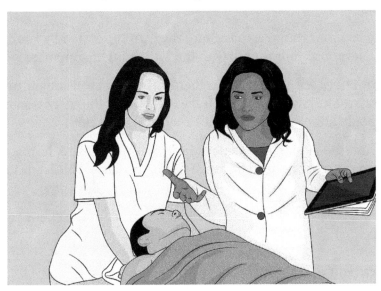

1. Vary things: The more techniques you have in your toolbox, the less chance of having repetitive motion on the same poor muscles. Go on more courses – expand your repertoire.

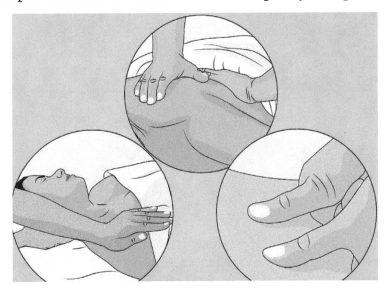

2. Know which techniques to avoid: There are many techniques commonly taught in qualifying courses that are best avoided altogether if you are intending to make a living out of massage. These include:

- Petrissage: "Open c closed c" – This technique uses the hands in the shape of a "C" to lift and push the tissues between them. This is very stressful to the thumbs, hands, and forearm flexors. There are many other ways of creating the outcome of this stroke.

- Thumb work: Most therapists have been taught to overuse their fingers and thumbs. Your thumbs should be thought of as the most precious tool you have. Only bring them out when absolutely necessary – approximately 10 percent of the time. Your forearms can do so much of your broad strokes and knuckles and elbows may be employed to get into the specific points.

- When you do use your thumbs, make sure they are supported by your loose fist or are flat on the body. Never use your thumb with the MCP joint unsupported.

- Effleurage with deviated wrists: Some therapists have been taught to massage the limbs with hands turned inwards to mould to the contours of the body. As far as possible, wrists and hands should always be kept in line or injury may occur.

- Effleurage from the side of the table: Many therapists learn to massage the back with strokes towards the client's head from the side of the table. This leads to unnecessary twisting and back strain.

- Effleurage from the head of the table feels just as good to the client and is so much better for your body.

Part 7. Incorporating Still Work

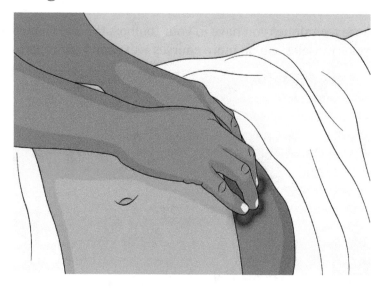

1. Include still work as part of the massage: It feels great. And it doesn't hurt your hands. Give yourself permission to spend time holding your clients feet, head, back, or anywhere you feel needs it.

- Focus and breathe energy into the area.

How to Maintain Healthy Boundaries as a Massage Therapist

Setting clear and effective boundaries can be difficult for many people, especially those providing health and wellness care. However, establishing healthy boundaries is a key for career success and life fulfillment in many jobs, especially massage therapy.

Steps

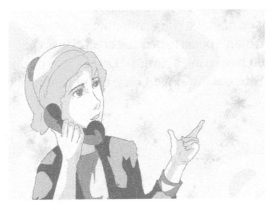

1. Establish clear boundaries from the outset: From the first contact via telephone, interview the client. Ask about their familiarity with massage, how often do they get it, what style they like, why they need one today. If you are getting a weird vibe simply state " I just want to be clear that this is a strictly therapeutic massage and that is what you are looking for." Be conscious of your own tone of voice, be firm and professional. Also, where are you advertising? make sure it is in a place and in a manner that cannot be misconstrued.

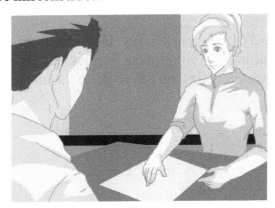

2. Once the client is with you, you can maintain your professional demeanor by having other professional procedures in place like an intake form that clearly articulates the professional standards of your practice.

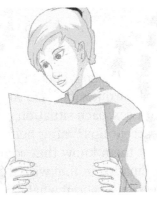

3. In your intake form, be sure to establish appropriate and inappropriate actions that a client may and

may not take. For instance: a client should tell the therapist if the pressure is too much or too little, a client should not say or do anything that is sexually suggestive. Additionally, consider this: because the pressure of the massage can turn on the parasympathetic nervous system and cause dilation of the blood vessels, it is common for a man's penis to become erect. This is perfectly natural and involuntary. While it is natural many men do have control over it. Learning to deal with these situations can also give men a chance to resolve any issues they might have about confusing touch with sex.

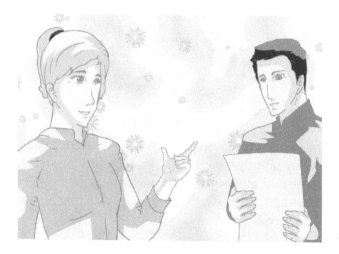

4. Make your intake form based on your personality: If you might have hesitation asking a client not to do or say something, putting it in your intake form can empower you. Later, if you need to ask a client not to do or say something, you can refer back to the intake form and remind the client of your policies.

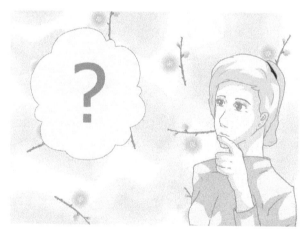

5. Learn to identify the signals and clues that a client is looking for sexual services. Address them directly if they arise. One example is the question, "Do you accept tips?" While this question rarely implies that they are only looking for sex, each situation needs to be looked at individually. For example, if the client asked "Do you accept tips?" after being touched near an erogenous zone, don't scream or run out of the room. Let them know that sometimes being touched results in sexual arousal but that you won't be participating in that with them. Too many massage therapists make the mistake of making the client feel guilty about what can be an innocent action. This does not, of course, mean they can touch you or say suggestive things to you.

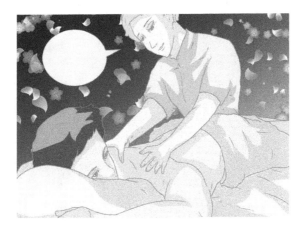

6. Don't let anything slide: Clients can feign innocence when you say something about it. A questionable comment or touch should be addressed as soon as it happens. One phrase would be, "This massage is strictly about me touching you, not the other way around. I will not continue if you do that again."

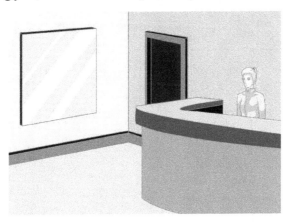

7. It isn't just about sexual boundaries: Setting boundaries also includes your policies and procedures around your business like cancellation policies, late fees/charges, no show policies which teach clients how you want to be treated.

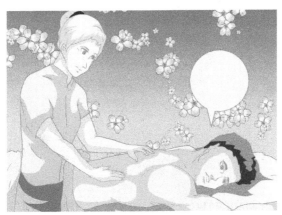

8. Boundaries also include things like active listening rather than always giving advice and how much you talk during a session -It is the client's session. Reassure the client that you have a non-disclosure policy.

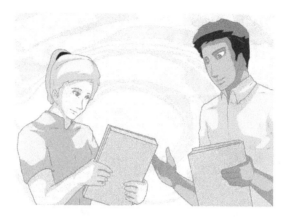

9. Boundaries also include things like having dual relationships with clients, having clients as friends, doing trades with clients for other services such as bookkeeping or legal advice. Keeping the roles separate is often the best for preserving the massage relationship although there have been successful friendships that originated in a therapist/client relationship.

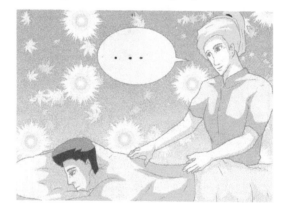

10. Keep your opinions to yourself about personal issues, religion, politics and the like. You are not there to judge a client's body, nor offer diet advice or smoking advice.

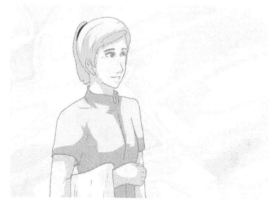

11. Transference and Counter transference happen. All relationships actually start with transference. What we are paid for as massage professionals is to be aware of our roles in these dynamics so that we can learn to not get hooked into crossing boundaries and preserving the therapeutic relationship.

Permissions

Index

T

Tendon, 42, 74, 92, 185

Tendonitis, 2, 42, 116

Torticollis, 2, 59

Treadmill, 55, 97, 109

Tumor, 3, 50

V

Vestibular Therapy, 2

W

Walker, 1, 77, 95, 109, 127

Whiplash, 86-87, 89, 91-92

Wound Care Therapy, 2

Printed in the USA
CPSIA information can be obtained
at www.ICGtesting.com
JSHW051355091023
49903JS00006B/156